MW01487839

praise for *sorry i keep crying during sex*

"*sorry i keep crying during sex* reads like your best friend's diary—a propulsive exploration of trauma, gender, and self with just the right amount of dark humor on top." **—Jen Winston, author of *Greedy***

"Do you think Taylor Swift knows there's an invisible string tying dementia, blow jobs, and 9/11 together? She might not, but Jesse James Rose definitely does—and after reading her memoir, I'm certain of it too. Rose wields words so incisively, always dancing the line between intellectual brilliance and delicious vulgarity with the ease of a silky hair flip. As tender as it is biting, *sorry i keep crying during sex* is an unflinching account of grief, identity, and reclamation in the age of Grindr and Wellbutrin. Rose folds memory and trauma into the pages of this book as deftly as she bakes pastries for her dying grandfather. A salve for survivors, a hand-squeeze for caretakers, and infinite awkward finger guns for sensitive queers everywhere—this book will hold you close and catch all your tears." **—Haley Jakobson, author of *Old Enough***

"A visceral, raw portrayal of trans and queer life, *sorry i keep crying during sex* will have you holding on for dear life. This book doesn't pull a single punch. Jesse Rose writes with exactly the type of tender, aggressive, in-your-face narrative gumption we need right now. Don't call it a debut: bitch, it's an *arrival*." **—Jacob Tobia, author of *Before They Were Men* and *Sissy***

"Sorry I keep laughing while reading *sorry i keep crying during sex*, but Jesse James Rose's darkly queer humor recognizes the absurdities of our lives even as we yearn and break and heal within them. Radical and fresh and giddily honest." **—Michelle Tea, author of *Against Memoir* and *Valencia***

"In a moment where trans and queer voices are more vital than ever, *sorry i keep crying during sex* by Jesse James Rose is a lifeline. With raw vulnerability and unflinching honesty, Rose has crafted a sparkling debut that is both achingly personal and universally resonant. This is not just a story of trauma, healing, and identity—it's a necessary reminder of how important it is to both be, and feel, seen. Through tender prose and bright insight, Rose gives voice to experiences too often silenced. We don't just need books like this one—we all need this very book." **—Eli Rallo, content creator and author of *I Didn't Know I Needed This*** "*sorry I keep crying during sex* is a nervy whirlwind of formal invention, overflowing with unforgettable lines. Only virtuosic comedy diva Jesse James Rose could morph a memoir of trauma, grief, and recovery into such a transformative blast." **—Henry Hoke, author of *Open Throat***

"*sorry I keep crying during sex* won't arrive wrapped in a bow, and it doesn't care about tidy endings. It is a vivid and vital account of what it means to navigate the world as a trans human, a survivor, and a caregiver all at once. It is the brutal poetry of healing in a precious and cruel world. It articulates the emotional whiplash of traversing some of life's sharpest dichotomies: being the target of unspeakable violence and making room for soft pleasure, accepting the final moments of a loved one's decline while resisting state terror at large, expressing yourself fully within the confines of a binary world . . . I opened the book while walking into the house, and I ended up standing at the door for hours because I couldn't put it down." **—Alyson Stoner, actor and author of *Semi-Well-Adjusted Despite Literally Everything***

"As a trans gen-z cusp, this book hit good and hard for me. *sorry I keep crying during sex* is a master class in vulnerability. Jesse answers our questions before we can even ask, and they take the reader places most authors wouldn't venture to." **—Dylan Mulvaney, *New York Times* bestselling author of *Paper Doll: Notes from a Late Bloomer***

"Rose writes with a wide-open heart and complete trust in the reader. A propulsive, provocative, startlingly candid work." **—Charlotte Shane, author of *An Honest Woman***

"Jesse's memoir is unlike anything you've ever read—a feat of experimental writing. It's hilarious, heartbreaking, beautiful, and raw (in more ways than one)." **—Zachary Zane, author of *Boyslut: A Memoir* and *Manifesto***

"If I was living through an apocalypse and needed something to burn for warmth and survival, I would choose this book last. *sorry I keep crying during sex* is full of feeling: pain, grief, hope, love. It grinded my heart to a pulp, only to put it back together again. Through it all, this book dissects identity with a beautifully manicured claw and ushers in a singular voice the world desperately needs. I would read Jesse James Rose's grocery list just to spend another second with her words." **—Nic Marna, @bookbinch**

sorry i keep crying during sex

a memoir

jesse james rose

abrams press, new york

Library of Congress Control Number: 2025937202

ISBN: 978-1-4197-7791-2
eISBN: 979-8-88707-459-7

Printed and bound in the United States
10 9 8 7 6 5 4 3 2 1

Some names and identifying characteristics have been changed.
Some dialogue has been re-created.

ABRAMS The Art of Books
195 Broadway, New York, NY 10007
abramsbooks.com

Well, you don't wanna hear about 9/11 . . .

—Mariah Carey

Author's Note

This book includes themes and mentions of sexual assault (including childhood sexual assault), grief, death, suicidality, 9/11, dark humor, PTSD, and brief graphic violence. You will never read a rape, though the subject is a through line.

This is my story of survivorship. I wrote much of this when I was my most mentally ill. I hope no reader finds those parts familiar, though I know many will. It has taken years of intensive therapy to even look at my own story, let alone write the rest. Not every survivor's story is compatible with mine, and if this isn't the right story for you at this time, I understand. This book will be here when, or if, you decide to return.

I dedicate this book to every victim, every survivor, everyone who knows what it's like to walk home on a midnight in October with a pain that words cannot describe. I hope this book can love you twice as hard as they hurt you.

I.

Thinking about that sex party I went to on the Upper West Side when I was twenty-two.

It was like forty twinks in their jockstraps and this guy Bruno fucked me on the king bed while everyone watched, dicks in hand, and he asked me if I wanted to try watersports and I thought that meant having sex in the shower so I said *hell yeah* and in the shower at this sex party in front of a barrage of onlooking horny twink strangers I learned very quickly that watersports is indeed not sex in the shower and as I wiped his piss off my face I thought yep this is my lowest point, it does not get worse, and I wished those boys would leave the bathroom so I could wash my face off but instead I put on my clothes and I walked forty-seven blocks back to Harlem with the wind turning his piss to plaster down my neck and when I got home I cried in the tub and wished my brain would break and I would forget everything about that night and they would all forget me and now I am twenty-five, I have not had sex in eight months, and I just cleaned my grandfather's piss off the bathroom floor again because he has Alzheimer's and his brain is broken and he can't even remember who I am sometimes.

I am 64% woman today, can't wait to be oppressed for this!

My best accomplishment of this season is this Pumpkin Cheesecake (Decorated with Walnuts and Sweet Whipped Cream Serves 6–8 *Click Here* to jump to My Recip—) where I messed up the pumpkin measurements and then I said screw it and started winging the rest of the recipe and my family said it was my Best Cheesecake Yet and I would like this to be a metaphor for the rest of my life.

What do you think your inner child would say if they saw you today?

Mine would say, "Is that a boy or a girl," and I would say, "That's the point," and then I'd get a lot gayer a lot quicker.

How far can corgis jump in the air?

At that same sex party I tried to do the cool move from the movies where you casually lean onto the chest of drawers and survey the array of limbs playing penetration twister on the bed in front of you and I saw some dust on the top of the bureau so I wiped it off onto the floor and this six-foot-five guy in a harness came barreling in yelling, DUDETHAT'SMYFUCKIN'COKEMAN, and it took me longer than I want to admit to realize I had brushed an entire line of cocaine onto the carpet.

My grandfather is singing to the birds again

Maybe it is time to try coke

Noon is absolutely not too early for cheesecake

Wait did anyone realize the coke dude misgendered me?

Why do all my friends think I'm cool enough to move to Brooklyn; I literally didn't recognize coke at a sex party how am I supposed to survive the JMZ?

Today my grandfather did not wake up soaked in his own urine and that is what we call a "good day" around here

The last time I was soaked in—never mind.

Guess who pointed out the same bird for the eighth time (hint: he is dying of a degenerative brain disease and is two generations above me)

Or is he one generation? How does that work

I'm calling my dad.

Ok, I just got off the phone with my dad

If I am diagnosed with Alzheimer's I am going to do one of those medically induced suicides where I go into the doctor's office and say, yes I understand the gravity of my situation, yes I know this medicine will end my life, yes I have my will ready et cetera, and then I will take the vial of death juice home with me and I will plan a huge family and friends weekend getaway where we all sit around and enjoy the ocean and reminisce on my illustrious career as a celebrated artist of the stage / screen / printed word and if I have kids they will be there and I will tell them how much I love them and I will feel an intense sadness for how much of their lives I will miss and I will have to trust that everything I was put on this earth to do I did to the best of my ability and it was enough and I'll remind myself that it only gets worse from here because one day the faces of my friends and my children would be unrecognizable to me and I would start forgetting where I am and what I've done in my life and my care would be exhausting for the people who matter to me and I love them too much to put them through witnessing my horrific decline into dementia. I will know I'm doing the right thing by letting this be their last memory of me and in a roundabout way I am taking care of them by dying then because it will be an honorable death and they won't have to spend years lugging me around to doctors' appointments and making me go through the old photo albums and breaking their hearts when I forget their names and I will save them the constant, unforgiving emotional labor of saying *it's not them, it's the disease* because at what point do we really believe that? So instead we will gather around the table and eat mac and cheese and cheesecake and go around the room and share our favorite memories of me and maybe I'll even invite a few of my lovers from over the years so I can look around and see my life before my eyes and who knows? Maybe I will feel some semblance of peace and gratitude and fulfillment. And then that night I will take the death juice and go to sleep and the next day will be my funeral and it'll be so convenient because everyone will already be there.

I'm calling it my Funeral Pregame.

"We treat sick dogs better than this," my uncle said after helping my grandfather into bed for his second nap of the day. He isn't eating this week.

Are you a bad person for wishing you could euthanize your grandfather?

Honestly so generous of me to plan my death, how convenient for all of you

Mental note: tell everyone to bring black to my Funeral Pregame

I wonder if Mr. Anderson will be free in fifty years to come to my Funeral Pregame

Talked to my therapist about my death plan, she said it was "interesting how I did not imagine having a partner."

Saw this Susan Sarandon movie where she gets diagnosed with something degenerative and literally invites her whole family over for her last meal and her own funeral—I'm so mad I thought this was my original idea, fuck you Susan.

What are we all wearing to my Funeral Pregame?

Are ball gowns—never mind

Finnegan did you ever love me?

The Fourth of July is coming up, can't wait to go to that bank on the East River where Finn and I watched the fireworks despite our mutual hatred for state propaganda and he told me to look up and a bouquet of electric sparks mushroomed into the open sky with every color I knew and he said that's what he felt in his heart when he kissed me and this year I will go there and watch the fireworks alone and cry not because I wish he never said that but because I wish I hadn't believed it

I just forgot if Finne/igan spells his name with an *E* or an *I* and I am too stubborn to look at his Instagram to find out.

I am going to find a way to make this his fault.

If you thought my absolute breakdown on the A train was impressive you should've seen what happened when that Troye Sivan song came up on shuffle when I was folding laundry way past my bedtime.

Can you have "nihilism with a lot of heart" or am I writing my own book genre here

Do you think my rapist has grandparents?

Some days I answer to he/him pronouns and sometimes I call myself a trans girl mind your own business

Are alt Twitters replacing Grindr these days?

Approximately how many dead Tomagotchis do you think there are

Are all the Tamagotchis in landfills or do they biodegrade

How the hell do you spell tomuhgahtchee asdkjfhja;

Does Finneaiougan have an alt Twitter?

Maybe I will invite my rapist to my Funeral Pregame

Hmm . . .

Like if he enjoyed the whole rape thing maybe he'd enjoy the me dying thing

OR!! He'd be all remorseful and sorry for the whole rape thing and either way I get the last word and I WIN.

If I can't be un-raped I can at least win

The only good thing about my maybe dying of Alzheimer's however many years down the road is I would forget being raped!

That doesn't feel like a win for some reason

I think we all know—

Wait this guy is totally doing watersports on his alt Twitter

I know a party he'd probably like!!

If noon wasn't too early for cheesecake then 11:00 p.m. is fair game for a second slice (I make the rules!!!)

Funny how these gays are tweeting and also so is my grandfather

Do you think the birds will know when my grandfather has died?

A List of People Who Should Be Grateful They Haven't Met Me in Person (Yet):

1. My rapist (but like, since the incident)
2. Finnegan (but like, since the breakup)
3. Finnegan's fiancé
4. My other ex's fiancé
5. The nurse I dated once's fiancé
6. DO WE SEE A TREND HERE
7. Mr. Anderson (more on that later)
8. Harvey Weinstein
9. All abusers, literally FUCK every abuser in this world
10. The inventors of Noom and Jenny Craig and whatever other fad diets are out there; you're ruining the lives of fat people and I hate you
11. The troll on my Instagram who started the whole "You Look Like Lord Farquaad" thing when I had a lob, I shit you not I cried
12. My former self; I was transphobic as hell and did not deserve rights
13. Idk cops???
14. Joanne
15. You know exactly which Joanne I'm talking about and we all should've listened to bell hooks when she told us that woman was a misogynist!!!!!
16. Where was I going with this
17. Oh, also God, or Jesus. I have notes.

Sometimes I wonder if the man who proposed to me when I was nineteen is alright

(He was not alright when I left him)

When does my gender stop being a "gotcha!!!" **finger guns** and an "I got your back, babe"?

Can I be over Finnegan and still hate his new boyfriend?

Or ~FiAnCé~ *as it is now*

(not me misgendering my ex's relationship, ugh).

My father called today to remind me what a saint he thinks I am for moving into his parents' house at the ripe age of twenty-five . . . how did I inherit such a good dad

For a long time I thought I wasn't gay enough because I didn't hate my dad

I love my dad

I also love daddies

These are actually not related statements!!

My dad drove up from Florida today and after seeing the current state of affairs with his dad and the birds and all, he said, "If I get Alzheimer's I am going to put a bullet through my head. I could never put you through this twice." I think tonight is the night I introduce him to the Funeral Pregame concept.

Should I make a PowerPoint about it or is that weird?

Fuck what if my dad isn't around for my Funeral Pregame

Or worse what if he is

I'm never having children that's final.

Despite the fact that I have not been to a gay bar in New York City in nearly a year (due to my sainthood) I still fucked like half the gay men there. I keep trying to come up for a word to describe this phenomenon but all I can come up with is "an absolute legend."

Should I move back to New York? This whole grandfather-death-thing might take a minute considering he was ignorant about the whole Funeral Pregame concept and I have decided I will not be forgiving him for this oversight

I want to move back but I can't because I'm afraid the moment I leave my grandfather will decide that's the moment to kick the bucket and I'll forfeit both my sainthood and my status as Beloved and Most Favored Grandchild

Spite is winning here because that's funnier than saying I stay because I love him.

Speaking of love, this twink I've been messaging on [redacted app] wants me to sneak into his apartment in the morning to wake him up and fuck him??

Sounds dangerous, I'm in

Wow he really did leave the door unlocked

Can you develop feelings for a twink in one hookup?

Why does my unlocked-door twink follow Finnegan on Instagram

Update: my ex also fucked my twink godDAMMIT can I get no peace

Some might call this "irony" or "coincidence" but they'd be wrong this is an UTTER TRAGEDY

Tragedy or travesty?

I'm not looking up the difference I don't care

Maybe that twink has an alt Twitter

OR Maybe I should've married that guy at nineteen

When he asked me, I shit you not he was mid flip of a blueberry pancake after our second sleepover in six weeks of dating (these are the exact statistics) and he looked up from the skillet in his short shorts and his glasses backdropped by his bookshelf of Neoclassical Portuguese Literature (he taught at Princeton, classic) and looked at me on his wooden breakfast nook bench where I sat next to his fluffy cat that made me sneeze and he said, "What would you say if I asked you to marry me?" and before I realized he was unflinchingly serious I said, "I don't even know your middle name!!" and he was very quiet for a second and so was the cat and then to make matters worse his head kind of slouched and he was trying to hide it but he couldn't because I remember distinctly his tears dropped onto the griddle by the blueberry pancakes and erupted in little tufts of steam and I must've come over to hug him because I will never forget sinking to the tile floor of his East Village apartment with a forty-eight-year-old man in my arms sobbing about how I was his last chance at love.

The weird thing was all his exes were dead too, which sounds spooky and here's why:

1. His teacher, died of old age (makes sense)

2. His former lover died in the AIDS crisis (sad)

3. His last boyfriend went off his meds and fell asleep in the snow

The third one is the sketchiest one to me but luckily Blueberry Marriage–gate happened to me in the summer and that gave me a modicum of peace (no snow).

If I fell asleep in the snow I couldn't have a Funeral Pregame

That would suck

If I did fall asleep in the snow there would be a whole media debacle (snowperson, not snowman!!!!) and I definitely don't want to ruin snowsculptures for everyone like that

Also, the frostbite thing would suck. I guess that's how he died? Either that or he got lost and collapsed in the snow of exhaustion and lay there for several days and got hypothermia or starved or something like that and died? I never got clarity on this

I also never got clarity on why Princeton-blueberry-pancake-Portuguese professor wanted to marry me after six weeks and two sleepovers either

I am going to tell myself it's because I am that charming and luscious

My grandparents got married at twenty

I very much would have married Finn at twenty-two if he asked me like he said he was going to but he didn't and now I am an unwed whore

My grandparents have been married for sixty-two years

Which is wild when you think about how the man who wanted to marry me was closer to the age of my grandparents' marriage than I was to his

Today my grandfather tried to eat a chess piece because he does not know the difference between objects and food and yet he still knows who his wife is and he remembers to tell her he loves her every night and that's just so fucked-up.

Do you think that man would've loved me if I tried to eat a chess piece after sixty-two years because my brain was rotting?

Or more importantly would he have still wanted to marry me if he knew I was trans?

Finger guns.

It's snowing, and I need to go to sleep.

Finn, After

Right before Finnegan and I broke up, we had sex.

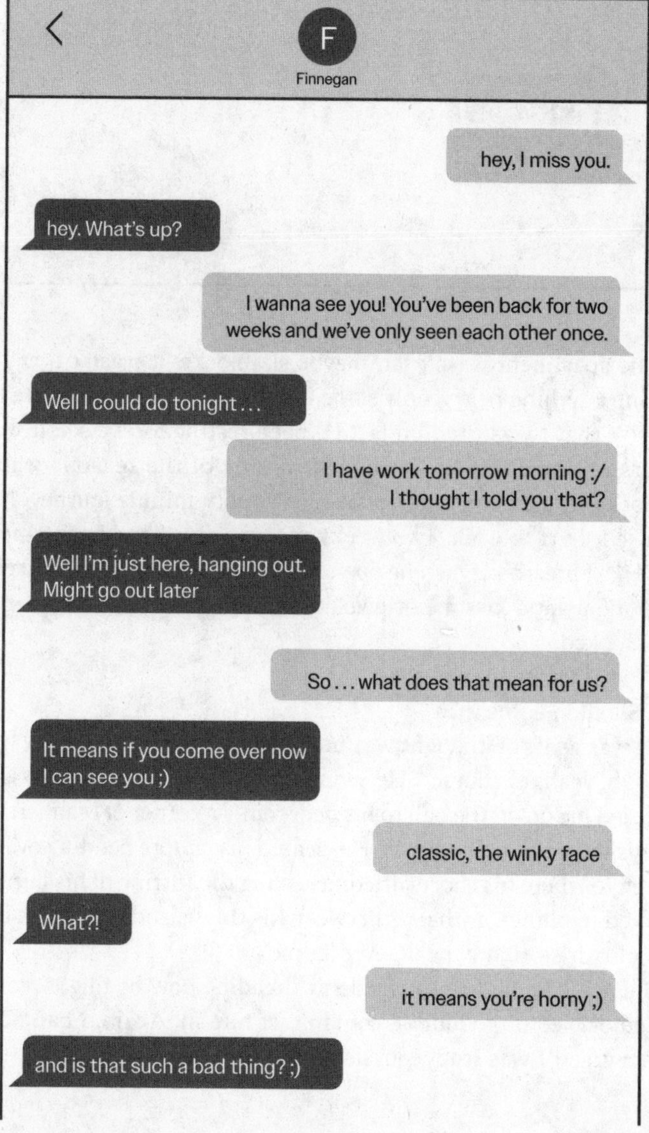

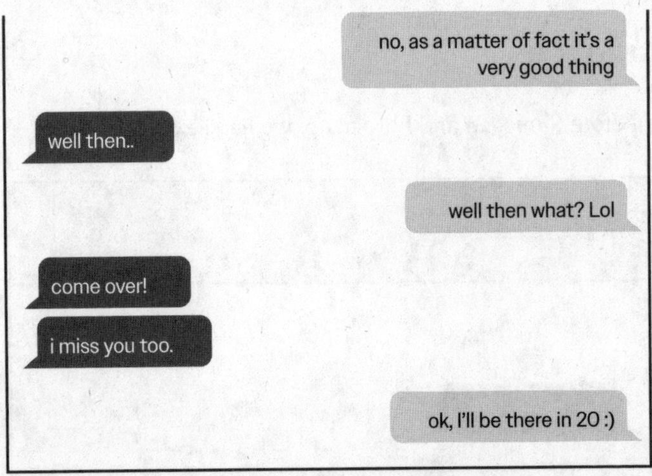

His apartment wasn't far, maybe six blocks. It wasn't that I was carrying anything heavy, only some extra towels and my favorite lube. It wasn't that I was tired; in fact I'd been resting for weeks. It wasn't blisters or dawdling or getting lost or any of the reasons walking six blocks would even consider being a twenty-minute journey. It was because it hurt to walk. Two weeks ago, you see, I had been raped.

"Hi," I breathed when he opened the door. I knew he would either scoop me up and kiss me or give me that usual smirk or tell me how cute I looked.

"Hey." He just stood there.

"Should I come in?"

It was as if the thought was brand-new.

"Oh, yeah, of course." He swung the door wide enough to let me in. He led me down the hall to his bedroom—a corner of Manhattan I'd only visited a select few times. He cleared his laptop, bending over just enough to where his shorts lifted, revealing the furring of his buttocks. I wanted to plunge my hands between his thighs and grip those blond tufts of hair so tightly he'd never let me go.

I unpacked my towels, suddenly dreading how he might react if I winced or bled or god forbid couldn't let him in. Again. I had no way of knowing if I was ready, physically, but I needed to try.

He didn't talk, he just slipped his cutoff sleeve jersey over his shoulders and danced out of his shorts. They slid down the fur and heaped at his feet, submissive to the thumbs at his waistband.

He turned on Troye Sivan's latest album, and I kissed him, my arms hooked behind his neck. I wanted him to be happy and to remember why he loved me. I started pumping his dick with one hand while I cupped his cheek with the other.

"Relax, babe. Slow down."

Embarrassed, I flirted. "I'm just excited to see you again."

He laid me on the bed behind us. I looked up at his blue eyes, framed by my legs on either shoulder. They were sharp, like melting glacier water and waxy cerulean crayons and baby boy hospital hats and warm dew. They were the eyes of the man who would take care of me and kiss my lips and fuck me like he means it and hold me after and say he was sorry for not texting me back last week. They were the eyes of the man who had chosen me over everyone else and was happy with that decision and still felt the fireworks from the Fourth of July even right now, even here. They were the eyes that would love me back to health and see all the things I couldn't and fix me. The eyes of the man who would never hurt me. My anti-rapist. My boyfriend.

Troye Sivan started into the chorus of *"I bloom just for you, I bloom just for you"* right at the moment my body seemed finally ready to let him in. If I wasn't so nervous about retearing or bleeding or how much it was going to hurt later, the irony might not have been lost on me. Finally inside, Finn smiled for the first time that night.

I watched his sharp melty glaciers roll back into his head.

"How does that feel?" I said the line I wanted to hear.

"Fuck, babe, you feel so good."

Somewhere in between the next chorus I saw his teeth peek out from behind his upturned lips again. He was happy. I wasn't in pain. My pelvic floor softened enough to make him moan.

"Oh, fuuuuck."

I was ok. He was inside me and I was ok and it didn't hurt and he loved it and he loved me and maybe everything was finally going to be alright. I was ok. I was ok. *Breathe.* I felt a tear slide out the corner of my right eye.

He looked at me, and I tried to turn my head, hoping he wouldn't see. It would be better if he didn't.

He took me by the chin, thumbing me back to center so I faced him. I could feel him harden.

"I just knew you were gonna cry." He grinned. "I just knew it."

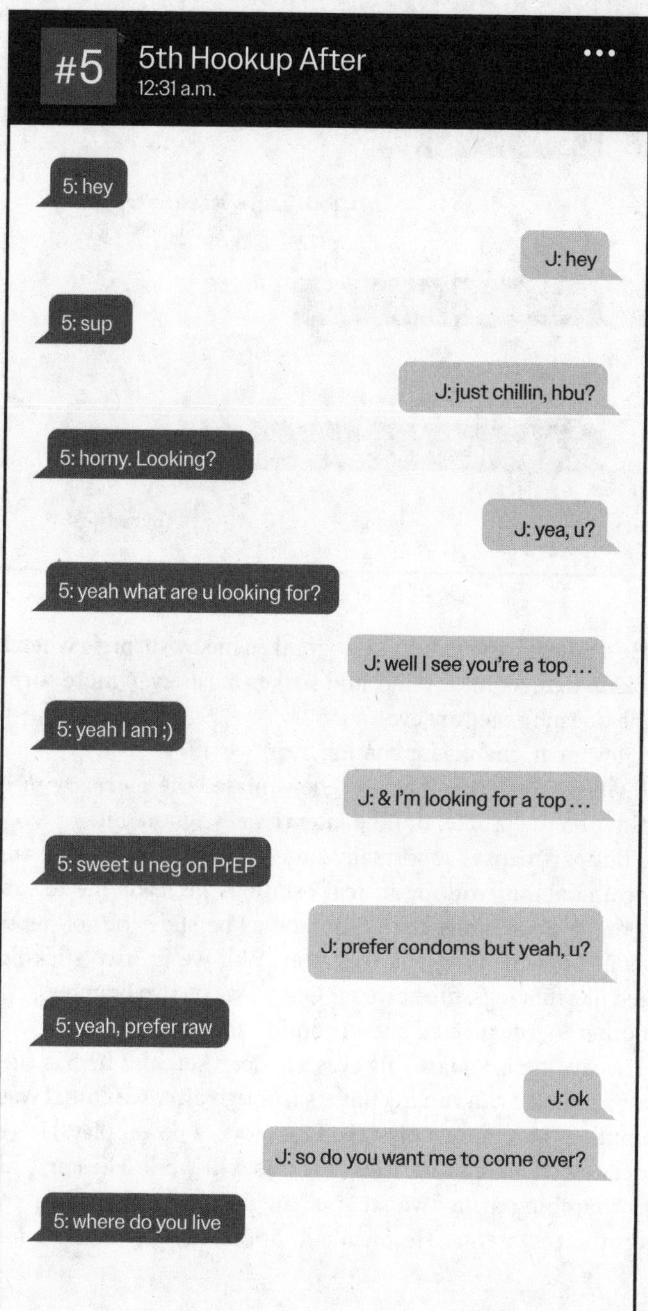
#5
5th Hookup After
12:31 a.m.
5: hey
J: hey
5: sup
J: just chillin, hbu?
5: horny. Looking?
J: yea, u?
5: yeah what are u looking for?
J: well I see you're a top . . .
5: yeah I am ;)
J: & I'm looking for a top . . .
5: sweet u neg on PrEP
J: prefer condoms but yeah, u?
5: yeah, prefer raw
J: ok
J: so do you want me to come over?
5: where do you live

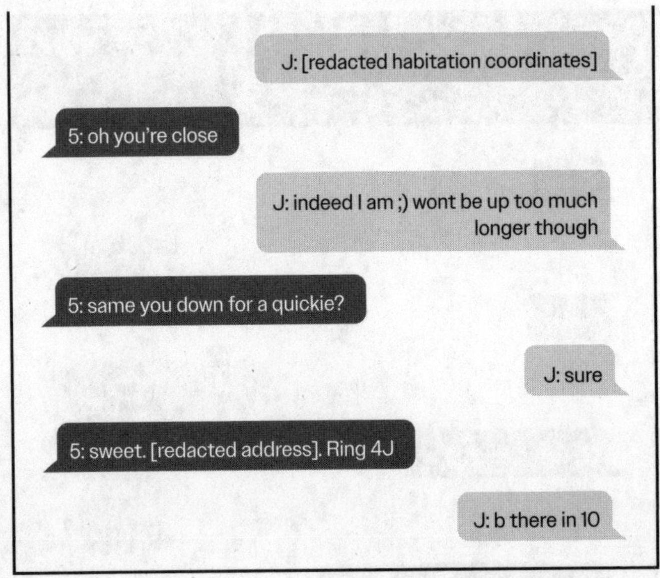

He's taller than I expected, so it takes me by surprise when I have to look up to meet his eyeline, and strikes me as even more surprising that he doesn't meet my eyes.

"Hey, man, thanks for coming over."

I wince, wondering if he somehow missed the *nonbinary: they/them* identifier on my profile, or if he intentionally ignored it.

The apartment is abnormally large—I comment on it, he answers something about working in real estate as he leads me toward the bedroom. He's skinnier than I am and as he slides out of his sweats I wonder how cuddling will feel after. Will we fit, two stick figures, stacked like flint logs, fire burning? Or will we be two brambles, sticking each other in unexpected and uncomfortable places?

His jawline is square, his eyes are deep set, and he has the kind of cropped hair I can run my fingers through after we cum. I waste no time pulling him in for a kiss, the first move, a power play. He's either dissociated or his lips are thin, but this will work. He starts kissing back, thumbing at my waistband, tugging my jeans down enough to cup their contents. He moans in approval—my favorite form of flattery—and I respond by kicking my pants down to my ankles. He returns the favor, pausing in between kisses to pull my shirt off, and then his own, revealing the hairless torso that caught my attention half an hour ago.

When he pushes me onto his bed (gray sheets, two pillows, *classic*) I can't tell if he's rough or just clumsy, but when he mounts the bed and pins my shoulders down I have my answer.

"Do you want it?"

The first words he's said since I put my mouth on his.

"Oh yeah." I punctuate the "oh" with a breathiness intended to get him harder. It works, I can feel it.

He's huge (the skinny stereotype exists for a reason!) and I silently curse myself for forgetting poppers.

"I might need those." I gesture with my eyes toward the bottle of RUSH on his bedside table. I follow it up with, "You're just soooo big." I manage to blush, and he hands me the bottle. I'm expecting him to grab a condom while he's at it and then I remember:

5: yeah, prefer raw

I remind myself this is fine, I'm on PrEP. I refuse to think too much about this being my first condomless encounter since Finn and I broke up. I remind myself I am not breaking the cardinal rule of our open relationship: no barrier-free sex with anyone else! We had decided sex without a condom was sacred, the pinnacle of intimacy, something only reserved for people in love. Like we were.

Were.

#5 has slipped a finger behind the fabric of my underwear, focused solely on my hole, and as good as it feels I know I do not love him. I decide not to argue with him about the condom; it isn't worth the risk of a refusal, another rape, and besides, Finn isn't my boyfriend anymore so the rules no longer apply. If I want to get over him, I might as well have the pinnacle of intimacy with #5 and #50 and #50,000 or whoever I want because then it wouldn't belong to Finn anymore and it would be mine.

Once #5 is inside me he is closing his eyes and moaning, and I remember why I love this feeling. My twenty-second high from the poppers has me begging for it *(deeper, harder, yes, fuck)* and #5 is loving it. The rough is welcome because it's in missionary and I get to watch him enjoy it and he is exactly the right size to shovel into my guts and dig Finnegan out because his dick reaches farther anyhow. I grope his ass (flat, but no matter) and push him in deeper.

He responds by grabbing my ankles and rocking me back for a better angle. I take another hit and I love sex and I love how #5 feels and I love how much pleasure he gets from me.

"I feel so connected with you." (I know, not my best line, but I was really feeling it.)

"Mm, fuck yeah." His eyes are closed.

"Are you good in this position?"

"Yeah, this is my favorite."

At his approval I lean back even more, arms out to the sides, perfect placement for a wrist-pinning, which he does. #5 begins breaking a sweat, which is hot even if annoying to dodge the droplets from his forehead landing dangerously close to my eyeballs. I've forgotten a spare pair of contacts so when he asks me to spend the night I'll have to sleep in these and I can't afford any preemptive irritation.

"I'm so close," he whimpers.

"Cum in me," I hear myself say because Finnegan wouldn't want that but Finnegan forfeited his right to want anything in relation to me so let's do this, #5.

We cum at the same time, which I hear is supposed to be romantic and sexy but truly it was a relief. In one move so coordinated I could only assume it was practiced he slides out of me and dismounts.

"Wow, damn," he exclaims as he disappears into the bathroom. I hear what I think is the faucet, and when he doesn't emerge after a minute I realize, to my horror, he's taking a shower.

I'm on his bed, cum spilling onto his classic gray sheets, alone. My insides hurt; nothing is where Finn left it. #5 has rearranged it to all the wrong places and instead of holding me while it settles, he's abandoned me to wash off any remnant of us. I feel used and small and overwhelmed. The distance between me and his shower is the distance between how I want to be cared for and what's actually happening, and in the overwhelm I begin to cry. I'm terrified he'll hear me because I can't control the volume and I can't turn onto my side to cry because if I do the cum will spill everywhere and mess up his sheets.

I grab a pillow and cover my face to muffle the sounds until I feel the cum puddles slithering toward his sheets. I have to clean up the cum so I can cry uninterrupted. I stagger, pillow in hand, to the kitchen, and pull a stream of paper towels. I shove the corner of the pillow into my mouth, a makeshift gag, so it muffles the crying and catches the tears while I try to wipe myself. I'm afraid the pillow will make contact with my abdomen and get soiled by the cum so I have to crane my neck and hunch my spine so the pillow hangs far enough away from my belly so I can get the right angle to wipe.

I'm suddenly fear-stricken with the thought that #5's shower could end any minute. I panic-hobble back to the bed, clenching my cheeks so nothing spills onto the ground. (I don't have enough paper towels for that.) I manage to stop crying and flip the pillow back under my head just as the water shuts off.

"Sorry, I was so sweaty, I had to shower." He emerges in a towel that hems at his ankles.

"Oh yeah, I get sweaty too," I assuage.

"Oh shit, man." *(wince)* "Did you wanna shower too?"

"No, I'm all good! I grabbed a paper towel from the kitchen to clean up the um . . ." I motion to my stomach, and the wad in my hand. "Where should I put these?"

"Uh, over there works." He gestures to a bin I somehow didn't see during my perfectly executed, complication-free paper towel retrieval.

"Are you a cuddler?" I ask on the way back from the bin. I'm afraid I've spoken a foreign language from the look on his face.

"A what?"

"A cuddler! As in, do you like to cuddle aft—"

"Oh, yeah, I don't really do that."

"Totally," I say, taking the cue and reaching for my underwear, my socks, my dignity, and the rest of my clothes before he can abandon me again.

He leads me to the door. I go in for a hug, undercutting his armpits with my forearms and he gingerly pats my back. I'm suddenly embarrassed I didn't ask him for the hug, breaking away and wondering how egregious a line of consent this is to cross.

I cover with "I really enjoyed that, you're super hot."

"Thanks, yeah, you too."

"See you around?"

He opens the door. "Yeah, I'll hit you up or something."

He doesn't hit me up. I don't "see him around." I barely see the first step outside 4J as my eyes well up with tears.

God, I'm so stupid.

"You live in New York!" My grandfather announces with an Appalachian twang on the last vowel, plucking a snow globe from the shelf and setting it next to him in his wheelchair. I remember when he bought the globe, on vacation with my grandmother at the turn of the millennium. It has fake snow and Times Square taxis and the Twin Towers are wearing little celebration hats. It used to sing "Auld Lang Syne" if you wound it up, now it just creaks like his wheelchair across the floorboards. I chase after him, cradling the globe and showing him where I live (lying, saying it's the South Tower, the only landmark he seems to recognize for whatever reason). I don't have the heart to tell him the towers are gone, or that he bought the globe for five-year-old me who wanted nothing more than to move to New York, who at twenty-five left the city to take care of him while he declines like the melody of the song over years of winding and winding. Snow globe Alzheimer's.

"Oh! Is that New York? Do you live there?"

Sometimes the worst part about having a rapist is not the being raped part, it's that he's genuinely hot.

This is in contrast to all my memories with Mr. Anderson, who was, in fact, ugly.

Ugly because he was a pedophile but also because he had a mullet in 2001 and not in the Hot Transmasc kind of way, in the child-predator kind of way, if there is such a thing.

Finn and I were literally in the same relationship and yet I ended up with PTSD and he is getting married how is this real?

One time in sixth grade I was on the morning show (back when I was straight and had bangs that neatly divided my goliath forehead in half hot dog style but like, before micro-bangs were a thing) and we would have the Word of the Day! segment and I was reading said Word of the Day! and the teleprompter I had to read off was tiny so I did my best to make out the tiny words and the entire school could see the Word of the Day! was "organism" (science week) but in my tiny teleprompter frenzy I proclaimed the word of the day was, I shit you not:

Orgasm.

You might think this is predictable but keep in mind I would have been twelve in sixth grade, and I didn't know what that meant let alone experienced one. Nonetheless, I spent the rest of the week being a disgrace to some and an "absolute fucking legend man yo Brock this is the orgasm dude!!!" to others.

You know, Mr. Anderson probably had an orgasm thinking about my plush seven-year-old body and that was before I was twelve so that at least counts for half, right?

The same month that I was molested was also 9/11

Who do you think had it worse

Look, I admit I have been sexually assaulted a lot but I have also made up for it by sleeping with at least 36 percent of the men in Manhattan so you have to understand my ratio of rapes to absolute bed-rockers is really good.

> Ok, I've only been raped once but I've been groped/harassed/stealthed/molested/assaulted/etc. more times than I care to count, I just wanted to write "ratio of rapes" because it's catchy.

You know what else is catchy? Feelings for your rapist—have I mentioned how hot he is?

Finn, Before

Maybe Finnegan didn't love me at all; maybe he was actually just mean.

I keep going over my relationship with Finn again and again—

Ha, Finn again. Finnegan.

Ugh.

Did you accidentally jack off to your rapist this morning or are you having a Regular Day?

Woke up to the first post on my Instagram feed being four hot boys in matching blue Speedos in Aruba or wherever and the one in the middle was my friend Magnus.

This Magnus is a friend I totally used to hook up with (back in my Top Era, you're welcome boys!!) before he got a job as a dancer on a cruise ship and of course at the sight of the Speedos I was immediately hard.

The closer I got to orga(ni)sm the more I zoomed in on the photo (leg hair! happy trails! dick prints!) and as I approached the Point of No Return I zoomed in on the third guy's face and I shit you not it was my rapist.

(Something I struggle with is how I have to call him my rapist, because it insinuates some sort of ownership that does not exist. He isn't mine. I do not claim him, he claimed me, and that was a lot of the issue. I need better words and better men, but for now I have neither.)

That is the story of how my pizza rose from the dead, and by dead I mean the depths of my stomach.

The best part is I did not have a chance to wipe my cum off my abdomen before my run to the bathroom, so while I was retching, my sperms were burrowing into the carpet on little egg-finding suicide missions.

In my defense he was wearing sunglasses so it was understandable that I didn't recognize him immediately.

My therapist said it was a good thing my sex drive was returning and I don't really think that was the point of all this.

I am going to post a picture of me in a Speedo looking hotter than all four of them and it will get more likes and I will consider this revenge.

I have now taken way too much time this morning to stalk each of the other three boys' social media (my rapist excluded, I do not need that algorithmic curse), and I have concluded based on the purely scientific criteria of comment interactions, who follows whom, and who has liked whose pictures, that Magnus is the only one who actually knows my rapist. I feel almost ashamed that I'm less worried about Magnus's safety and more angry that they seem to be having a good time in Aruba or wherever.

Their post has 313 likes, which is a record I can surely blow out of the Aruban or wherever waters.

It is now 312 (I made some decisions).

My Speedo post already has 98 likes in ten minutes. I can taste this victory already and let me tell you it tastes better than half-digested pizza rocketing across my taste buds in reverse.

Please do not psychoanalyze my need for sexual validation in the face of seeing my rapist I am fragile right now it would be more useful for you to grab the Shout from under the sink because the cum isn't coming out of the carpet.

Much time later I would learn the series of events that led up to that photo from someone else working on the same cruise. Though he didn't know my relationship with my rapist, he happened to know the whole story.

It wasn't as bad as I thought—Magnus had invited my rapist onto the ship with one of his guest passes. When my rapist arrived, he met another boy, Kyren (the slut of the cast so I'm told and I respect it). My rapist fucked Kyren, and then Magnus found out about it and it became a multiweek spat between Kyren and Magnus. (Very

"You fucked my guest!" "Well he wanted to fuck me and you weren't back yet!" "You don't own him!!" and so on.) Both of them had been fucked by my rapist, but the hang-up seemed to be the order of events, and the right to the fucking. Sex dibs, if you're familiar.

This situation fascinates me for multiple reasons:

1. Kinda legendary of my rapist to be such a catch that multiple boys are fighting over him long after his guest pass expired.
2. Kinda fitting that my rapist seems to leave a trail of destruction wherever he goes, including the middle of the ocean.
3. Kinda wild to learn my rapist is, in fact, capable of consent.

I've been stalking Kyren's Instagram for weeks now ("fieldwork" I've been calling it, the scientific alternative to "coping"). He's a classic rave twink: bone skinny, nineties chokers, lets his thongs peek out of his low-rise jeans paired with captions like "It's warmer inside ;)." He is a constant invitation for, dare I say it, objectification.

Is it still objectification when you intentionally position yourself as an object? I should know, I did it for years with my own thongs and Instagram captions when I was pretending to be a boy.

That's what gets me; Kyren is a lot like I was years ago. The brunette coif, the angular jaw, the innocent face, the "hi, daddy" doe eyes. Mine are prettier but despite this we both are/were the ideal cocktail of promiscuity and boyhood. Look up the "please, sir" emoji and imagine it on a twink, you'll get the idea.

I wonder if Kyren's brazen eagerness translates off-screen to a real-life desire to be fucked into oblivion, and if that's true did it shield him from being raped by my rapist? What I mean is, was there a moment during the fucking where Kyren asked my rapist to stop or slow down or switch positions? And did my rapist listen? Or did they never get to that point?

I wonder because the inherent risk of communicating your needs and asking someone to stop/pause/adjust/change/etc. during sex is it immediately puts you at the crossroads of Rape and Not Rape. If they do stop/pause/adjust/change/etc. they have chosen Not Rape and the alternate is obvious. But if you never ask someone to stop/pause/adjust/change/etc. during sex you don't reach those crossroads. And if you're just more open to whatever is going on because you are, say, sex-starved-at-sea you might not ever reach those crossroads the way I did on a fateful midnight in October.

By that logic, is it possible that Kyren never asked anything of my rapist because he has different boundaries or interests (especially after days upon days in the open ocean with no physical touch) and never asked my rapist to stop? Does that make it Not Rape by default because they never hit the crossroads? If I was more desperate or sex-starved-at-sea, would I have not asked my rapist to stop, thereby never reaching the crossroads myself?

I had fucked so many men before my rapist that I had lost count. Hundreds—and I mean hundreds—of situations where I asked people to stop/pause/adjust/change/etc. and every single one of them chose Not Rape. It's also possible other people hit those same crossroads with my rapist but in those instances he chose "Not Rape." This doesn't really apply though to the current situation because Kyren might've ruined this for all of us by not reaching the crossroads and we'll never know whether my rapist is a Serial Rapist or a Selective Rapist.

I know there are a lot of people (especially sex workers) who will be mad at me for saying all of this because it rubs dangerously close to the implication that being sexually adventurous or posting slutty Instagrams is "asking for it." I know—believe me,

I know—that isn't true, and even through Kyren posts thong pictures it's not appropriate to objectify him. All I'm saying is that it's possible Kyren's sex drive and preferences might've shielded him from an assault. We can't rule out the possibility that my rapist just wants what he wants and if it aligns with you, you're lucky and you don't get raped, and if you don't align then . . . you do.

Ironic for me, the nonbinary, to be creating a binary.

Kyren looks like the kind of guy who loves to get his guts wrecked in doggy (this is a compliment because it is the sluttiest position, arguably, and the hardest one for me). My rapist and I stayed with missionary because the placement of my asshole works better for this and that meant that I got the distinct pleasure of watching him assault me, and I hate that it helps me to imagine Kyren as just another hole to my rapist so he fucked him in doggy so he wouldn't have to look at him but he raped me in missionary because he wanted me so bad that he had to have me and I'm pretty to look at.

I am so jealous of Kyren I could die.

There is a correlation between desirability and rape-ability and apparently I'm at the nexus of both for my rapist. And by this logic that means it is possible he liked me more than Kyren.

I am so jealous of Kyren I could die.

Is it bad that I almost hoped that my rapist had assaulted someone else? Kyren, Magnus, someone on the ship? I don't *really* wish that but I don't want anyone else to have good experiences with him so long as mine is what it was. I prefer him as either celibate or a Serial Rapist because if he's a Selective Rapist then I have to thumb between Kyren's posts and Magnus's posts trying to find reasons they are less assaultable than I am. Another binary. I'm stuck.

It is more convenient for me to think this way than to accept that my rapist didn't care a whit about me and has since learned to care, and now everyone else (Kyren) is getting the sex treatment I deserved. It is more convenient for me alone, but that's how it is these days. Me, alone.

Last night, I'm embarrassed to admit, I jacked off to one of Kyren's pictures. It was one of the thong ones and in my fantasy I was fucking him in doggy and he was loving every second of it. And then Magnus found out and was pissed at both of us but we didn't care because there were no guest passes or sex dibs and with fucking that good Magnus's opinion doesn't matter anyway.

Weird how in my fantasy we never hit the crossroads. Perhaps that was on purpose.

What I do not want to think about is how it's possible that Kyren did indeed hit the crossroads of Rape and Not Rape and my rapist chose Rape because he is a serial fucking rapist and now I've just done to Kyren what everyone seems to have done to me, which is tell me I was asking for it because I was being a whore.

Do I owe Kyren an apology?

(Don't answer that.)

My Speedo pic is clocking in at 2,741 likes. At least there's that.

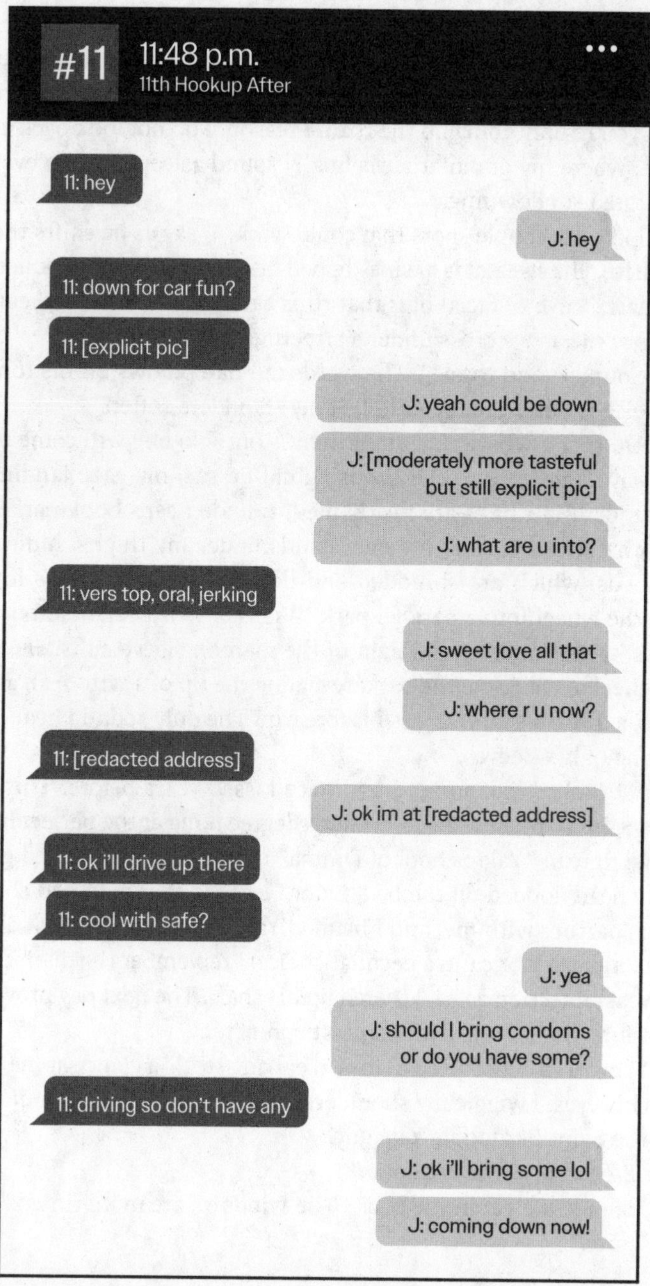
#11
11:48 p.m.
11th Hookup After
11: hey
J: hey
11: down for car fun?
11: [explicit pic]
J: yeah could be down
J: [moderately more tasteful but still explicit pic]
J: what are u into?
11: vers top, oral, jerking
J: sweet love all that
J: where r u now?
11: [redacted address]
J: ok im at [redacted address]
11: ok i'll drive up there
11: cool with safe?
J: yea
J: should I bring condoms or do you have some?
11: driving so don't have any
J: ok i'll bring some lol
J: coming down now!

"Hi." I smile breathlessly, securing my hair with an elastic and closing the car door in one coordinated swish. It's not dangerous to get into a car with a man you don't know at 11:48 p.m. on a weeknight when you're only going up the road, I reason. I do not look back at my house, where my grandfather is finally sound asleep after an evening of agitated sundowning.

"I know a couple spots that could work," I say as he shifts the car into drive. His sweater is a wine-dipped raspberry, deep hues pulled out by a dark brush of facial hair that runs ear to ear. A diamond earring winks at me as we cross under a streetlight.

"Sounds good to me." The words fall like pillows off his tongue. His voice is buttercream and I feel my shoulders soften.

"Up there, where that streetlight is out. No one will come down this way." I gesture to the snoozing cul-de-sac, my gaze landing on his hands. #11's nails are neatly filed, rounded caps bookmarked by smooth cuticles. I slide my own hands under my thighs, hiding my nail beds, which are shredded and flecked with scabs. His fingers coax the wheel into a parallel park. Wisps of hair peek out about his wrists, tamed under the weight of the maroon sleeve cuffs. He turns the wheel to complete the park, revealing the tip of a tattoo; an arrow, a line, a directive lane across his forearm. The only sound I hear is the shifting of his sleeves.

#11 looked like a man I had once kissed years before. This man had a Saint Berdoodle and a master's degree hung at the perfect height for me to read "Yale School of Drama" in upside-down bolded gothic as my head flopped off the bed. Later I learned that man had cheated on his partner with me, and I blamed Yale for the Drama of it all. He used lotion as lubricant, a peculiar choice. I remember the distinct fear of a yeast infection as he lathered up his shaft. The next day proved no yeast infection, but a distinctly soft sphincter.

"You're so cute." #11's diamond earring steals a glance at me along with his eyes. I wiggle my shoulders in affirmation. He really did look like the Saint Berdoodle Yale guy.

"Stop, you're the cute one."

"Should we get in the back? The windows are more tinted."

"Sure."

We make eye contact as we pull our pants down next to each other in the back seat of his car. Moonlight splashes onto the pale of his thighs. Our legs are so long, or the back seat is so narrow, that my leg clamps over his, interrupting the moonlight. He squeezes the inside of my hamstring as I stroke myself. He cups the back of my neck with his manicured fingers and leads me down between his legs.

I ready him with my mouth, hand him a condom from my pocket, and tangle myself in my jeans as I attempt to turn around for him.

"One second." I manage to stuff the condom wrapper in what I think is my pocket as I pull off my shoe and free my left leg. Doggy is not my favorite but the options in the back of a car under a streetlight at 11:54 are limited.

"Do you have any lube?" I've forgotten mine.

"No, but this will work." He lifts a bottle of Lubriderm from a bag in the passenger seat. I don't have much time to think before his lotioned tip begins to press. The momentum pushes my head against the window, and he begins. I feel the hem of his sweater tickle my lower back, and I arch so it swings above my lumbar. He thrusts faster and my cheek presses harder against the window. The glass is cool, pressure is soothing, the fog of my breath evidence of the pleasure.

"I'm about to cum—" He pulls out, rips off the condom, and for some reason I mouth dive onto his dick. The liquid salt swirls against the remnants of rubber and Lubriderm, and I swallow before the taste sets in. His eyes roll back, his thighs quiver, and he gasps for air.

"Christ, that was hot."

I want to kiss him but I'm afraid of the advance being rejected especially after a mouthful of semen. I settle for burning the memory of his orgasm in my mind, something I caused, something I achieved. He pulls a wad of napkins out of the same bag as the lotion, offering me a few.

"Do you wanna cum?"

I want to lay on his chest in the moonlight on the top of the car while planes pass overhead and planets burn and he adorns my neck with sweet nibbles of desire but I settle for getting fingered while I sploosh onto the napkin he armed me with.

"Damn, you're just . . ." He runs his filed fingernails across my stomach, tracing the divots between the muscles. ". . . so fucking sexy." He punctuates with a fleeting moment of eye contact, still erect, still not kissing me. "Your hole is perfect, too." He retracts his hand and sinks against his side of the car. The diamond earring's back clicks against the window.

"Thanks, you're really hot yourself. That was really hot." My voice is lower than I expect. I sit up, beginning to untangle my jeans from the footwell.

He squints. "You look familiar."

Ok, so I was right. It was him. I decided not to take the usual "oh, maybe social media?" approach, since he is almost definitively the guy from years ago who cheated on his boyfriend by inviting me over to get railed with his master's degree as an audience. My shoulders tense.

"Yeah, I was thinking the same thing. Have we . . . met before?"

"Nah, I was in a relationship for years."

"Oh, I thought for a second you were a guy I hooked up with like, a long time ago."

"Oh yeah?" He chuckles, tucking himself back into his pants. The fog has obscured the windows. His earring doesn't twinkle with the movement.

"Yeah, but this guy had a dog, and I don't see any dog hair in your car, so . . ."

"What kind of dog?"

"I don't know the breed." I pretended to search my brain. "But he was some kind of doodle, I remember that."

He looks at me. "Do you remember anything else?"

"Only that his master's degree certificate was the biggest thing on the wall." I force a laugh. "That guy went to Yale, if I remember corr—"

"Is this some kind of joke?" His words are sharp, a nail file on a papercut.

"No, not at all, you just look like that guy, that's all."

"Well." He leverages silence. "I'm not that guy."

"Totally." I shake my head. "Sorry for being weird and bringing it up, it was really the lotion that did it. That guy used lotion as lube, so did you, I've never seen anyone else do that before. You definitely have a doppelgänger, in looks as much as lubricants."

Reading the room—or the car, rather—I open the door, turning around for another apology before leaving.

"Hey," he says without meeting my gaze. His sweater slouches on his shoulders. "I would appreciate your discretion with all this."

"Dude, we just fucked in a car, do you think I'm gonna tell everyone about this?"

"No." He winces. "I would just . . . really appreciate your discretion."

"Ok."

"Ok."

"Sorry for thinking you were someone else."

"All good." He waves it off. I am about to shut the car door when his phone buzzes. The screen lights up revealing a photo of two people, one kissing the other's cheek, and between them, a dog. I can't see it well enough to identify the breed.

#11 pockets the phone, and then looks at me.

"Nice to meet you tonight. You okay to walk home?"

"Yeah, it's just down the street."

I shut the door, turning around only to collide with the neighbor's trash can. I mutter some obscenity before fishing out the condom wrapper from my pocket. My hands return empty. I look up in time to see his headlights turn out of the subdivision, condom wrapper in tow somewhere in the back seat. I open my phone to find him on the app so I can warn him about the wrapper, but the chat is missing. He had blocked me and driven away.

I storm back into the house, tears brimming, aching to collapse on my bed and not wake up till the morning. I stifle my cries as I lock the front door behind me, terrified I'd wake my grandparents.

"Who's there?"

I freeze, turning slowly to see a figure perched in the center of the kitchen. Moonlight from the window dances off silver wheel spokes, hiding the shadowed figure of my grandfather in his wheelchair. I exhale.

"It's me, Grandpa, it's me." I sleeve my tears away and kneel beside him.

"Oh!" He cracks into a grin. "James! Where have you been? How's New York?"

"I wasn't in New York, I was just outside. Can I help you?"

"Oh, I don't need any help. I'm just fine, thank you."

It occurs to me I have no idea why my grandfather is alone in his wheelchair in the kitchen in the middle of the night. I hear the faint sound of water running in the bathroom. My grandmother must be awake, washing something. Perhaps he had another fitful night's sleep resulting in an accident and she had to put him in his wheelchair to clean the bed, and he managed to roll himself into the kitchen.

"Are you having difficulty sleeping, Grandpa?"

"No, I'm just waiting for breakfast."

The oven beams 12:13. "Breakfast won't be for a few more hours, you should really go back to sleep. Can I take you back there?"

He isn't looking at me.

"Grandpa?"

Still, he stares off. I cross his line of vision, preparing to repeat the question.

"Oh, hello!" He grins again. "You're James! I remember you. How is New York?"

I want to answer. Instead, I slip behind him, redirecting his wheelchair toward his bedroom. The wheels *eek* across the floor as the tears come back. At least someone remembers who I am.

A List of Affirmations I Am Trying Out:

1. Loneliness is temporary
2. Everything is easier with a deep breath
3. Consent is mandatory and it is ok to ask for this
4. My body is a temple
5. Grief doesn't go away, we simply grow around it
6. Gwyneth Paltrow is a victim of the system too
7. It's ok if you don't really believe #6
8. Wealth inequality really does cloud our judgment on these things, don't dwell on it
9. Escapism is a valid trauma response
10. God grant me the serenity to accept the things I cannot change, the courage to change the things I can, and the wisdom to know the difference
11. Honestly that last one doesn't feel right but I tasked myself with writing ten of these and I'm really running out here
12. It wasn't your fault
13. Someone else is gonna love you, you just haven't met them yet
14. #7 can also be applied to #12 but it doesn't make it any less true

The phases of Alzheimer's are outlined two different ways: one with three stages, one with seven. Both are generally agreed upon by experts in the field as accurate ways to characterize the course of the disease, though I find one more helpful than the other.

The three stages as outlined by Johns Hopkins University are:

1. Preclinical Stage
    - This isn't technically a stage; it denotes how the brain begins changing long before symptoms surface.
2. Mild, Early Stage
3. Moderate, Middle Stage
4. Severe, Late Stage

With respect to the Johns Hopkins folks, I don't find this particularly helpful, especially considering the "Moderate, Middle Stage" encompasses everything from having difficulty with logistics to hallucinations, which feels too broad a spectrum to assign a single category, especially when you consider this is where people with the disease spend the most time.

I prefer the seven stages as outlined by Dr. Barry Reisberg, and not only because we share an alma mater, nor because his last name sounds quite similar to a 2023 Best Actress nominee whose appearance on the ballot was both controversial and exciting, but because they make the most sense.

The seven stages as outlined by Dr. Barry Reisberg's Global Deterioration Scale are:

1. Normal (no cognitive decline)
    - Remembering everyone's name and only a PET scan would indicate signs of cognitive decline.
        - *Example: When you are twelve and your grandfather takes you to Barnes & Noble every time you visit because he says books are the window into understanding the world and he wants you to understand it.*

2. Very Mild Cognitive Decline
    - Presents similarly to age-associated memory impairment.
        - *Example: When you are eighteen and visiting for the holidays and your grandfather forgets where he put his keys, which literally everyone does.*
3. Mild Cognitive Decline
    - Cognitive impairment characterized by difficulty following conversations, or short-term memory loss.
        - *Example: Last year when you are playing Up the River, Down the River with the whole family and your grandfather has played out of suit twice in a row, which is frighteningly uncharacteristic for the reigning family champion of two decades.*
4. Moderate Cognitive Decline
    - Defined by mild symptoms of dementia, or significant loss of mental function.
        - *Example: Sometime during this stage we discontinued my grandfather's phone because he couldn't figure out how to work it and it felt compassionate to alleviate him of this frustration, especially considering how difficult it was for him to carry on a conversation if someone called him.*
5. Moderately Severe Cognitive Decline
    - Difficulty managing tasks like choosing outfits or remembering their phone number or address; moderate dementia.
    - Most people at this stage will be able to eat, bathe, and enjoy mostly independent daily routines.
        - *Example: My grandfather is in a wheelchair so he does not have quite the same experience. In fact, we cut out half a wall in the primary bedroom so he could fit the wheelchair around the corner and we gutted the shower so he could transfer into the shower seat unobstructed.*
6. Severe Cognitive Decline
    - Unable to remember most events (with the exception of childhood memories), delusions, hallucinations, mood changes.
        - *Example: My grandfather asks every day when we are going home. He has lived in this house for nearly three decades.*

7. Very Severe Cognitive Decline
    - Significant help eating, swallowing, sitting up. Most communication is nonverbal.
        - *Example: Sometimes I feel guilty for wanting him to advance to this stage faster so our tenure with this misery is shortened.*

Every time something new happens, like when he forgets a name of a family member or doesn't finish his plate of food or asks when we're going home, I consult the steps. While I understand each case of Alzheimer's is unique, it helps me to get a sense of his progression. It is comforting to know at least one of our declines is clinically outlined. His mental deterioration is predictable and patterned; I'm losing my mind without direction. Less Reisberg steps, more like a plummet into a bottomless pool.

Finn, Before

"It's because you're so big!" I teased. He rolled his eyes.

"Shut up." He crawled on top of me to kiss me, sliding the pillow out from under my hips. He had placed it there for easier access and "a better angle." I didn't care what angle so long as it involved him and his floppy blond hair and a day's stubble and no alarm the next morning.

"I'll get you in eventually, I promise."

"I'm not worried," he said, returning the lube bottle to the nightstand where it wouldn't get swept away in the comforter. Another kiss. Another, another.

"How are you still hard?" I tugged on the evidence.

"Because you're hot"—*another*—"and I like you"—*another*—"and I get hard just looking at you"—*another, with tongue.*

"I want you inside me so badly . . ."

"And we'll get there!" Sensing my frustration, he reassured me with a thumbstroke across my cheek.

"I really don't know why I'm having such difficulty . . . I like, never have this problem."

More men than I cared to count had entered with ease, my body an enthusiastic receiver. Why was it faltering now? He had attempted to soothe me with his tongue. It felt fantastic, but when he replaced his tongue with his tip my body seized and we were back to square one.

"Maybe it's because you're gorgeous and you look like an Abercrombie model and I want you to like me and I'm nervous? Because it's our first time?" I sat up so we could be eye level. "I'm sorry, I really want this to be special and I feel like I'm failing."

"Hey now," he said, "you're not failing." I wrapped my legs around his waist to sit on his lap. Finn locked his fingers together behind my back and put his forehead against mine.

"I like talking to you, hanging out with you, I like kissing you, I like going to dinner with you, I like you. I like your brain, I like the way you think, I like that you're annoyingly right about everything. I absolutely want to have sex with you. Like, deep, passionate, fuck-your-brains-out sex better than any other guy you've ever been with and it's ok if it doesn't happen tonight. I just want to be here with you, whatever happens."

"Why are you perfect?"

I learned my eyes were leaking when he thumbed a tear from my cheek.

"I'm not, but maybe we're perfect for each other."

Then it started: the waterworks, the tears, the crying.

"Hey, hey," Finn started, and I managed another apology before really losing it. My shoulders started to heave and my body began to shake. I shuddered trying to hold it in, trying not to be That Insane Girl, bargaining with my emotions to quell long enough so I could make love with this boy and his melty glacier eyes and his coiffed hair and his Abercrombie abs and his chest hair and his inexplicable attraction to me. But trying to stop it only made it worse and I collapsed onto said Abercrombie shoulders and gave up. I sobbed. It hurt. I sobbed more.

"Baby, it's ok. I've got you." He held me tighter, open palms, cupping the curve of my rib cage as it throttled between cries. Somehow this only made it worse because he was trying to tell me it was ok, that he liked me, but it wasn't "ok" I was being Insane and no one actually likes this. My tears pooled in his clavicle and I realized this was probably it. He would make up an excuse to go spend the night back home and if I was lucky I'd get the text the next day that he had a good time the past few weeks but he just wasn't feeling it. This was the end, the Insane Girl in me managed to fuck it up before he could even fuck her.

Finally my eyes ran out or my body was too tired and my breathing evened. He disengaged the hug with a look of concern I couldn't bear. I dropped my head.

"Are you ok?" he asked. "Did I say something that upset you? I'm so sor—"

"Oh god no." I swallowed. "That's the thing, you're doing everything right and it all feels like a dream and that's like . . . painful? I don't know, maybe I'm being crazy right now."

He took his hands to either side of my face. I saw the little lines around his eyes I would learn only wrinkled when he concentrated or cared or was thinking.

"If this is your crazy, I'm here for your crazy. It doesn't scare me or make me like you any less. I'm crazy too."

“Not crazy like this!”

“No, definitely not like this.”

“Oh, shut up!” I laughed, a welcome relief.

“You’re the most beautiful person in the whole world to me. Crazy and all.”

Whoever created the image of love as an arrow piercing the heart must have seen this moment. Or at least known what it would feel like. The arrow doesn’t pierce you because you’ve been struck or hurt or shot down, it’s a representation of how they see you: straight into the heart. They have laser precision right into the thumping beast in your chest where they witness the ugliest parts of you hemorrhaging black-and-blue fireworks and they decide to stay there anyway. The symbolism made sense. Finnegan made sense. I took the arrow in my chest and pressed it against his, kissing him, hoping it would pierce his heart and no matter where we went the arrow would always connect my heart to his.

“I want you inside me,” I said, and I meant it.

“Yeah?” he said.

“More than anything.”

And then he was, and it was perfect, and I loved him.

A List of People I Want to Meet:

1. My foster children. When I have enough money I can buy a big house in a nice place with lots of rooms and then when children who have been assaulted or are kicked out for being queer or trans need a home, I could give them one and we can work toward reunification and maybe I could make one of the hardest parts of their young lives a little easier, who knows I'd have to meet them first
2. An anti-rape activist who was also once a rapist
3. Cate Blanchett
4. That trans woman who won the longest *Jeopardy!* streak; I think she's fabulous
5. The Dior people. I would like a dress.
6. The Twitter gay I followed last night (yum)
7. Osama bin Laden
8. Future me, I gotta know how this ends

Something fascinating about 9/11 is that a lot of people make it a "no fly" day now but I was not afforded that luxury when I was seven because Mr. Anderson fully said the equivalent of "yes, fly" by unzipping his fly in the back room of the music classroom and showing me his dick.

Fifteen years later, a professor said he lived by the words "the enemy of my enemy is my friend" and I asked him, a queer man in his fifties, if he thought the oppressive state government in America was his enemy and he said, "Yes."

(For the record, I agree.)

I wrote my final paper in that class about his philosophy: The enemy of my enemy is my friend. My thesis was that if America is his enemy, then Osama bin Laden must be his friend.

(The reasons for this should be obvious.)

I received an "A" with a "meet me in my office" scrawled in hasty red pen underneath.

I did not meet him in his office. I think this has more to do with my molestation trauma than the opportunity to defend my intellect.

Should I send him a copy of this book? "Sorry I missed office hours, hope page 49 makes up for it."

I titled my paper "Love Letter to Osama," and honestly if more people had written love letters to him maybe he wouldn't have fallen down the religious-extremism-to-global-terrorism pipeline.

Some people are going to criticize me for "humanizing a terrorist"; let me remind you that while y'all were busy with terrorism and being racist about it, I was getting molested, so thanks a lot.

Something inhumane about the whole U.S. Navy SEALs killing Osama bin Laden operation is that they literally shot him in front of his kids.

Like, his daughter was there and she was, according to reports, under the age of ten. One of the SEALs who spoke Arabic made her identify the body. I'll say it: She did not deserve that. It's not her fault about the whole towers situation, she was literally not even born when it happened.

I on the other hand was seven, and you know what happened.

Have you ever met a gay person who didn't like a good 9/11 joke because I sure as hell haven't!

The United States spent an unbelievable amount of money trying to find Osama bin Laden so they could murder him.

I guess the Hague was not fit for him? Unclear. He was very tall.

I was obviously not on the planning committee for all this (see detail: ten-year-old daughter).

A Nonexhaustive List of Things the U.S. Government Spent Money On for the Whole *Kill Osama* Mission:

- Guns
- Backup guns
- Sixty million dollars' worth of helicopters and planes
- Average salaries of $54,000 per Navy SEAL (based on 2011 Department of Defense Data)
- Multiplied by the number of SEALs (twenty-three, at least) that's around $1,242,000, but I'm sure there were more over-seeing training, processing paperwork, buying planes, guns, and backup guns, and the fact that this particular team likely

had salaries closer to six figures each, so easily $3,000,000 of SEAL salaries

- Boots, gotta be at least $250 they look SLEEK
- Camo jackets, $50 each, though I found thrift sites where you can get 30 percent off with a valid military ID, which I am assuming said SEALs have or we have bigger issues at stake here
- Four-Tube night vision goggles valued at $65,000 each
- An entire life-size model of the compound Osama was reportedly hiding in built to scale in North Carolina
    - This has since been destroyed; I looked into it as a potential location for a book signing. The marketing team has informed me that even if it were standing today it would "not be prime for photo ops."
        - I can only assume they mean the lighting is bad.
- Band-Aids, $12.88 for the Family Adhesive Variety Pack at the CVS on Twenty-Third and Broadway
- Penicillin shots (Navy SEALs get syphilis too!), $54 per shot at pharmaceutical market rate
- There was also a dog, and while I don't know how much the dog cost, just knowing there was a dog to pet on this helicopter gives me comfort. Kinda like how my rapist had candles. It's the little things.
- More guns
- Zip ties, $24.04 for a ten pack (if they went through the same Minnesota-based eBay seller I'm looking at)

Imagine how much all of that cost, and now imagine if we had reallocated like, 10 percent of a single helicopter's worth of money to offering therapy to, I don't know, victims of childhood sexual assault.

> But we don't, because it's more fun to kill people in a state-of-the-art Chinook bought with working-class tax dollars than it is to kill the rape culture we live in. That's the American dream, baby!!

I like to tell people at parties that when the Navy SEALs executed the mission and flew over to Pakistan to kill Osama they literally crashed one of their little planes into the side of his compound.

A lot of people attributed the crash to the Pakistani mountain's weather being particularly turbulent and they had no way to simulate this during training, but I would like to invoke an old patriotic adage and say, "God's timing is always right."

We could also say something about karma here but I don't think this is the time for pitting religions against each other seeing as how that got us into this mess in the first place depending on who you ask.

Another fun fact is the actual killing took like nine minutes but they were there for forty securing all the other inhabitants of the compound including his wives and other children (this is where the zip ties come in).

They also shot Osama bin Laden so badly that his face was reportedly unrecognizable. The SEALs decided the best way to confirm the body's identity would be through his height. (It may surprise you to learn that Osama bin Laden was tall—six feet four to be exact.) Now, in all their preparation (recall the list) the Navy SEAL admiral who oversaw the mission forgot a tape measure, so he did the next best thing:

He asked one of the younger SEALs, "How tall are you?"

And the young SEAL answered "Uh, six feet two, sir?"

And then the Navy SEAL admiral made the young SEAL lie next to Osama's dead body to confirm that the body was, indeed, roughly six feet four.

Please imagine you're like, twenty-two, on your first big Top Secret Global Murder Mission with twenty-two of your strongest, hunkiest friends, at least one of whom brutally shot a man in the face in front of his daughter, and you have to LIE DOWN NEXT TO THE CORPSE.

What was going through his mind while he did that? I have to know.

> Like, how close did he lie? Was he inches away from Osama's arm? Was he on the ground, or in a plane, or in a truck? Was Osama's body still leaking fluids at the time from the whole murder part? Was he in a body bag, or did he have to be taken out for accuracy of the measurement? Did the SEAL close his eyes? What did he smell like? How long did he lie there?? Did anyone take a picture for their records, or just look at it and go, "Yeah, guess he's about six feet four, must be Osama! Thanks for your help, Jared."

When they all got home President Barack Obama awarded the Navy SEAL admiral with some medal and then presented him with a tape measure on a plaque, ad-libbing something about "don't forget this next time."

Don't tell me war criminals don't have a sense of humor!!!

I do not know how my college professor felt about this, we haven't spoken.

Do you think that young Navy SEAL was gay?

Maybe he needs an insane trans girl with trauma for a partner; if anyone has his number let me know.

Another reason I'm interested in this SEAL (I have named him Jared for simplicity's sake and because I feel like that's a solid Navy SEAL name, Jared) is because he was quite young during this mission in 2011, and that means he had to be REALLY good at being a Navy SEAL. Like, they're not taking the dregs of this specialty Marine force on the *Kill Osama* mission so this guy has the kind of prestige I'm looking for in a man.

"Jared, and James the Hot Trans Girl" (sung to the tune of Jared: The Galleria of Jewelry).

Navy SEALs also have big biceps and I think that might make Finnegan jealous.

I wonder if Jared also got a medal? Seems like the least they could've given him after he lay down next to a bleeding smelly global "mass murderer" corpse that might not have even been in a body bag.

Jared is also probably pretty hot, come to think of it. Hot in like, a non-patriotic kind of way. In an "I chose to have this crew cut" way. In an "I can bench you as foreplay" kind of way. In an "I would never vote for a Republican after marrying you, babe!" kind of way.

Reminder that Jared is literally six feet two (yum).

He's also probably around my age because if he was in his early twenties in 2011 he's roughly thirty-six now and that could work.

How do you think Jared feels about, say, antifa?

Are the enemies of Jared's enemies his friends, and if so, who are those people?

Do you think if Jared lies next to me in bed he will get flashbacks? In my defense I am not six feet four.

Maybe he also cries during sex because of his PTSD, and look, at this point trauma bonding might be a promising place to start.

Last fun fact I swear: Did you know they dumped Osama bin Laden's body in the ocean because no country wanted to claim it?

I relate to this because Finnegan dumped me.

Conspiracy theorists have oft used this as "proof" that America didn't actually kill him and he's very much alive and well. I just think that's so uncreative. How we could be using that time to, I don't know, advocate for victims of childhood sexual assault.

(Yes, how antifa of me!!!)

My uncle was a first responder on 9/11 (he is very much alive and well) and when I was in college they were building the memorial. My first New York 9/11, there were two gigantic, parallel blue beams in the sky made of light, symbolizing the towers. I kept looking out my dorm window that night wondering how on earth they found lights that big and that bright, thinking it must be part of the memorial at Ground Zero, and maybe I could find the light source there. When I arrived downtown, I found the construction site locked, and the blue beams still a block away. Moments later I had snuck into the adjacent parking garage and, thanks to the friendly security guard on duty, found myself on the roof across from two unthinkably massive lights saddled in their cases. I still have the picture I took. It comes up on my phone every year.

I never told my uncle about this; I guess that was my way of silently paying respect to his service. 9/11 must've affected him deeply because he never talks about it, in that way a lot of men never talk about what they so desperately need to be talking about. There is light out their windows too, but they can't look for reasons I've stopped trying to understand. It's as if they are locked in a snow globe where the music no longer plays.

Now that it's fully constructed, I visit the 9/11 memorial every year. I'm always astounded that instead of keeping the blue lights it has been memorialized as a vacuous pit with water hemorrhaging from all sides plummeting into a gaping, bottomless hole.

It's not the irony of the plummeting or the terror at the sight of the pit that gets me; it's that out of everything I've seen in the world that memorial is the only thing I've ever found that encapsulates how it feels to be sexually assaulted.

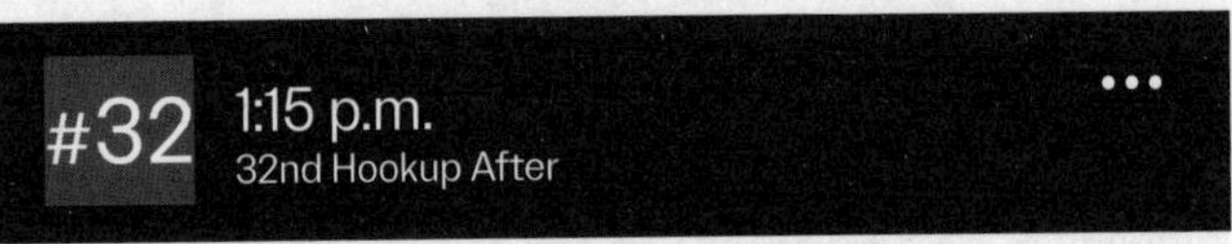

I'm in the sauna at the gym and I'm definitely not looking at the Daddy next to me.

He is doing the Straight Man thing where he can't complete a Figure 4 stretch and I am doing the Gay Whore thing where the corner of my towel barely covers the tip of my cock. Both of our towels splayed so our bare hip flesh is locked in the staring contest our eyes can't have. His body hair forests down the side of his thighs—massive slabs of muscle, the watermelon-crushing kind. If I look at them any longer the blood will rush down and pop the towel off my tip. I avert my gaze.

#32 is sweating profusely, and I'm waiting for him to gather the towel from his lap and wipe his face so I can see underneath where the forest thickens. He's bald like Vin Diesel and cut like George Clooney and I'm ready to have his children. There's another man in the sauna, some dudebro in a pair of swim trunks listening to a podcast. If only #32 would wipe his face.

You might think this is invasive to look at #32 this way, but you have to understand there are signals:

- Open towels
- Splayed legs
- Sparse cock coverage
- A quick ball pull with eye contact
- Excessive body rubbing and touching
- Stretching that exposes yourself
- Stretching that allows you an excuse to look at someone else
- Looking around more than usual
- Mirroring the other's actions, affirmatively coded as YES, I AM GAY TOO, show me the goods

So far #32 has displayed two of them. Well, technically one and a half. His towel is only half-open, and while he is stretching, I can't tell if he's stretching to stretch (straight) or stretching to give me a better look (gay as hell). Usually I need at least three items from the list to confirm, but if I've gotten one and a half signals and haven't given him one, he'll have no incentive to continue. I offer him Mirroring the Other's Actions by sliding my right ankle over my left knee and folding effortlessly, hoping he'll take my limberness as proxy for eagerness. He glances over; his eyes are hotter than the sauna stones. He counters by switching the legs of his stretch.

That's a full two signals, so it's my turn. Dudebro in the swim trunks has his eyes closed, oblivious to the homosexual mating ritual taking place before him, so I'm free to respond. If I Mirror again and switch my own legs I'll expose my too-hard dick and then I'm in dangerous territory. Instead I choose to add a spinal twist to my Figure 4, employing Stretching That Allows You an Excuse to Look at Someone Else. #32 responds by shifting in his seat and hiking up his towel. Is this a third signal or a comfort movement? He begins to twist away from me when I see it: his shaft snaking out, peeking onto the wooden bench. It twitches, and to my delight I watch it harden and lift back into the forest. Stretching That Exposes Yourself. Third signal. *Booyah.*

By some miracle (one I absolutely deserve!!) dudebro in the swim trunks stands with all too much noise and leaves. Now it's down to me and my not-so-straight Vin-Diesel-Clooney-Forest-Daddy. He looks over again, this time for longer. I try to smile but I can't hold his gaze. Was he staring me down (hot) or scaring me off (comp het)?

I readjust my towel. *Abandon ship.* He flicks yet another glance, so fast his eyelashes barely move. *Ok, maybe not.* I take a leap of faith and go in for the Ball Pull (sans eye contact). In my periphery he reciprocates, pulling his own. *Oh, hell yeah.* Unmistakably, Diesel-Clooney Daddy and I are gonna fuck.

We begin to fool around in the sauna, which is always a fright because the risk of interruption (or banishment, humiliation, jail) is high. Any sexual activity is a workout, but even the CrossFit world champions would have to train for aerobic fucking inside the swelter of the sauna. I, defending champion, have stolen a few grabs at his cock, he's moaned, he's called me "good boy," which I'm deciding is not gendered because that's convenient right now and I am more worried about whether he's gonna have a sexuality crisis and bolt.

He does stand, but instead of bolting he turns to me.

"Fuck, baby," he whispers, despite the sauna being nearly soundproof. He keeps staring. I keep being hot. "I want you."

Thank god. "I want you too."

He closes his hand around my throat, and I assume he's going to push my head down between his legs (where I belong!!!) but instead he picks me up by the neck.

"Come with me."

He's taking me to the shower where I will have his children.

The shower stalls in this gym have dark blue curtains, which is ideal for cruising because you can't see who's inside. The first shower could be dudebro, the second vacant, the third a business executive rinsing off, the fourth where #32 has me pushed against a wall with his hand pulling the bun on the back of my head.

In that same fourth stall #32 has pushed the shower nozzle away from us, the water lukewarm. I imagine this is because he is also a climate activist who doesn't want to waste (1) water and (2) time not pleasuring me.

And pleasure me he does. I am returning the favor, crouched underneath him when he shoots into my mouth. A rope of semen splatters into what I think is my eye, and I am about to reach for the nozzle to wash it out when the sting of pain never comes. In fact, as I move, the semen splatter moves with it and I discover, to my horror, that I am wearing my glasses.

"Fuck, baby boy, that was hot." He bites me on the chin, hard.

"I can't believe I was wearing my glasses this whole time," I joke, and he grins.

"That's why I didn't turn the water on hot."

"Huh?"

"That's why I didn't turn the wat—"

"No, I heard you, what did you mean?"

#32 nips at my ear and slides a hand around to grab my butt. "I didn't want your glasses to fog up." He pats a cheek, and slips out of the stall.

I collapse on the bench, semen gobbed on the corner of my mouth, and wonder why this is the nicest thing a man has done for me since I can't remember when. That probably explains the tears that come. At least, I hope it does. I want to run after him and ask for his phone number and his address and if he has a dog and whether the second shelf of his medicine cabinet is spoken for already, but instead I grab the shower handle and twist it past the bright red temperature strip. Within seconds steam fills the stall, clouding my lenses, holding me in a fog of warm loneliness. I cry and pretend I am sweating instead.

Finn, Before

I did not care that it was humid because I was sitting on a park bench with Finnegan eating ice cream. Despite being sexy and in demand, I had never been on an ice cream date before and Finnegan was the perfect person to go on an ice cream date with because he was who I wanted to be around the most. Finn nursed the chocolate side of a combo cone while I tongued the rim of mine, forbidding anything to drip onto my shorts. I believed I had successfully funneled a tongueful of rainbow sprinkles into my mouth when I felt them rain on my inner thigh.

"You are a catastrophe." We both laughed.

"And you love it."

"I do." He kissed me until I heard a plop on the bench slat.

"Oh, that is soooo your fault!"

He shrugged, and I wiped the ice cream off the park bench with a recycled napkin and skipped over to the trash can. I was mid victory pirouette when Finn asked me what on earth I was doing.

"Making art." I punctuated the melodrama with ballet arms.

He tried not to giggle through his latest mouthful. I began a pattern of lunges and head bobs that would put Julia Louis-Dreyfus to shame. I added guitar sounds for good measure, and at a particularly high set of *neer-neer-neer*s Finn broke into a laugh, vanilla droplets dribbling down his chin. His cone was unguarded, so, I took my chance. I bit off the top.

"Oh, you're bad!" He licked my own cone before I had a chance to react. Sweet victory; we were even.

I upped the ante with a finger to his swirl, plucking an even swatch of flavors and lifting my finger to my mouth. At the last second I swiped it across his nose. He looked at me in a way that makes me wonder whether he was going to eat the ice cream next, or me.

He slid his free arm around the small of my back. I was on high alert—was he going for my cone? His cone to my face? What was his strategy? He looked me in the eyes, his melty glaciers dripping at the rate of our dessert in the humidity.

"You think you're gonna win this?" he teased.

"As a matter of fact, I think I am."

"No way."

"Way!"

"No. Way."

I take a lick. "Way."

He looks at me like dessert is the last thing on his mind. "Babe, it's not even a competition. I won." He kissed me, vanilla and chocolate and arrow-through-the-heart pink.

"How's that?" Sprinkles, arrows, daggers, hope.

"Because I have you."

I am scraping the oil off the roasting pan when my grandfather wheels himself out of the bedroom and into the kitchen all bright and chipper and full of life, despite being somewhere near the end of it. He greets me with a resounding, "Good morning, what's for breakfast today?" It is 5:58 p.m. and I have set the table for dinner.

There is no rule book for how to respond to this. I've checked. There are, however, two options:

1. I can save him the embarrassment of being wrong about the time of day and attempt to pass off veggie pot pie with deviled eggs as breakfast foods and take the chance that his memory has already ctrl-alt-deleted all information regarding morning meals because if it hasn't the confusion could lead to agitation and sundowning and a distressing night for all of us involved.
2. I can correct him and say it's nighttime and explain that he's just had a nap and it's time for dinner and then his first interaction upon waking is the dignity-stripping realization that he's wrong.

I rack through my list of affirmations (the ones I could barely write ten of), searching for anything that might guide me toward a response. Unfortunately for me, there was nothing to the effect of "it is impossible to protect your grandfather's feelings and maintain your own sanity, this is how degenerative disease works, it is not your fault," but unlike the rest of my affirmations that one doesn't fit on a quaint Instagram graphic so I guess the omission is understandable and indicative of a larger cultural issue around the pop psychologization of wellness that I don't have time to get into because I need to give him an answer.

I place the roasting pan on the drying rack and run my wet fingers through the dish towel as I make my way over to him. I bend over to give him a hug.

"I have food for you over here; are you hungry?"

He wheels over to the table where his pot pie portion sits steaming.

"Yes, as a matter of fact I am!"

A List of Reasons My Rape Doesn't Count:

1. He wasn't a stranger and everyone is raped by strangers in alleyways
2. I met him on Grindr, which is supposed to be a fun place
3. The blood vessels under my eyes didn't burst from choking
4. My hymen wasn't broken
5. I wasn't drunk
6. I'm not in a sorority
7. I wasn't beaten
8. He wasn't taller than me
9. He wasn't a psychopathic predator who stalked me beforehand for months
10. He didn't break into my house
11. He didn't wear a ski mask
12. He didn't have a knife
13. I'm not a troubled girl who lost her parents in a tragic accident at age fourteen and got in with the wrong crowd and became addicted to opiates
14. He wasn't in a gang
15. He's hot
16. I told him I wanted to have sex with him
17. He didn't have a bunker in his house
18. He didn't spit on me
19. He used lube
20. He wasn't my uncle
21. He wasn't my brother's friend I had been dating
22. I don't go to Catholic school
23. I'm not pregnant
24. He had candles, which was a nice touch
25. I never had to pick him out in a lineup behind a two-way mirror
26. My SANE nurse didn't have a clipboard and a bedside manner
27. They didn't take pictures of the marks on my body and the prosecuting DA played by a pretty white actress with a power bob didn't tell me they would "get him, whatever it takes"
28. He doesn't have a criminal record

29. He didn't tie me up
30. He didn't blindfold me
31. He didn't cut off my left ring finger
32. He didn't steal my underwear
33. He didn't force me to shower at gunpoint
34. I don't live alone in a corner apartment you can see into from the street if you're driving a white pickup truck between the hours of 1:18 and 4:46 a.m.
35. It didn't happen in the middle of a gay club
36. He said he liked my smile
37. It didn't happen in a janitor's closet
38. It didn't happen in a dungeon
39. He didn't use power tools to—
40. He didn't read the police textbook on Rape Forensics to stay six steps ahead of the police the entire time
41. He didn't sodomize me with various household objects
42. He didn't drive a nail gun through my temple
43. He didn't bludgeon me with a lamp from my bedside table
44. He didn't leave my body in a ditch
45. He didn't dismember my remains in his bathtub afterward and clog the drain with chunks of tissue causing a pipe to burst over apartment 6B
46. He didn't threaten my life
47. He didn't turn himself in after
48. He didn't flee the country
49. He didn't solemnly swear to tell the truth, the whole truth, and nothing but the truth
50. He didn't film it for his buddies
51. It didn't happen in the stall of the men's bathroom
52. It didn't happen in the stall of the women's bathroom
53. He didn't have an accomplice who guarded the bathroom door
54. His friends didn't write letters about what a good guy he is and publish them online
55. His friends didn't cyberbully me
56. He didn't cover my face with a pillow
57. He wasn't even that aggressive, come to think of it
58. He didn't spike my drink

59. He didn't give me drugs
60. He didn't follow me home after work
61. He didn't offer me a ride in the rain
62. He sent me nudes and they were at good angles, which shows he cares
63. I didn't scream "rape"
64. I didn't scream "help"
65. I didn't bite his penis off and swallow it so he would be forced to check into the hospital and be caught by Ellen Pompeo, who carried it around in an organ transplant cooler all day
66. He didn't gag me
67. He didn't bind various parts of my body
68. I don't have big blue eyes that make me look innocent and young
69. I wasn't underage
70. He was wearing light blue boxer briefs and they never wear those; they always wear boxers or nothing under their jeans
71. He didn't have an identifiable tattoo on his lower left calf
72. He wasn't my boyfriend who was known to have a mean streak
73. In fact, he has a lot of people online who post about what an amazing teacher he is
74. I wasn't held hostage
75. I wasn't a prisoner of war
76. It wasn't in the upstairs bedroom of a frat house with all my friends below
77. It didn't involve a famous Hollywood producer
78. There wasn't a trial
79. He wasn't investigated
80. There wasn't sentencing
81. They didn't "get him back" in jail
82. I wasn't left in an alley for dead
83. I wasn't told I was "lucky to have survived that"

These are all things that happened to other girls when they were raped on *Law and Order: SVU* and *Grey's Anatomy* and *Baby Reindeer* and *Unbelievable* and Jodie Foster in *The Accused* and theirs counted,

I think.

A List of Reasons It Does Count:

1. I said no.

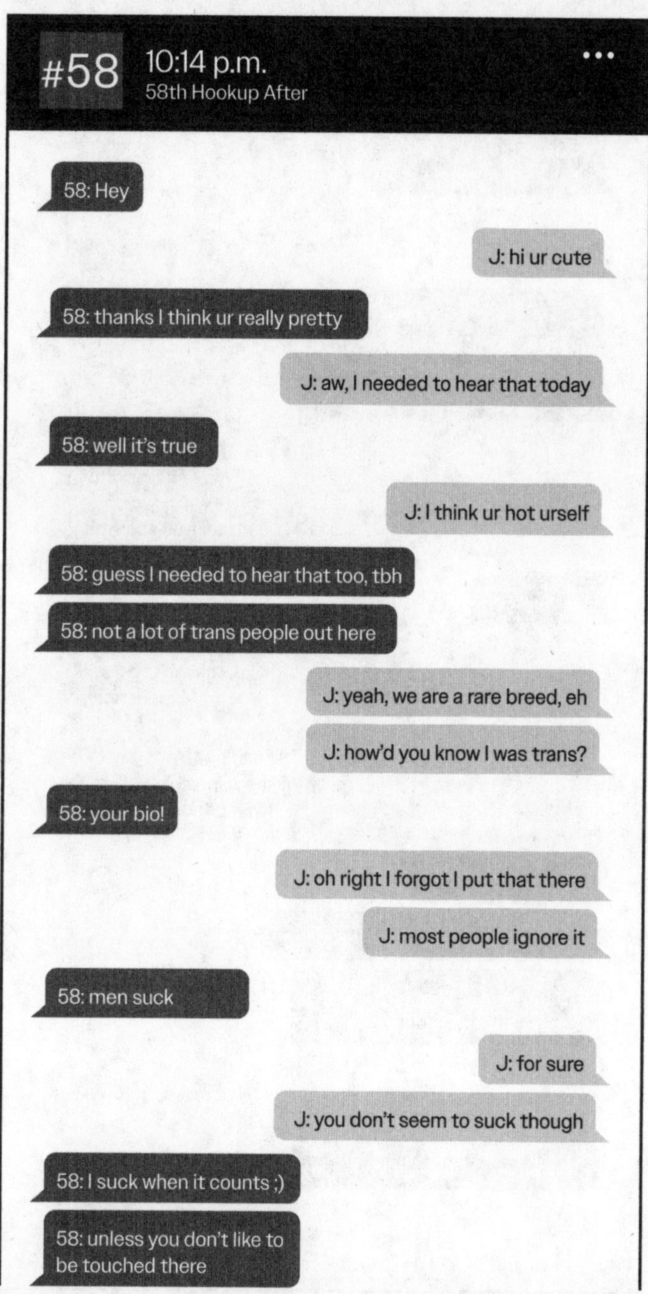
#58
10:14 p.m.
58th Hookup After
58: Hey
J: hi ur cute
58: thanks I think ur really pretty
J: aw, I needed to hear that today
58: well it's true
J: I think ur hot urself
58: guess I needed to hear that too, tbh
58: not a lot of trans people out here
J: yeah, we are a rare breed, eh
J: how'd you know I was trans?
58: your bio!
J: oh right I forgot I put that there
J: most people ignore it
58: men suck
J: for sure
J: you don't seem to suck though
58: I suck when it counts ;)
58: unless you don't like to be touched there

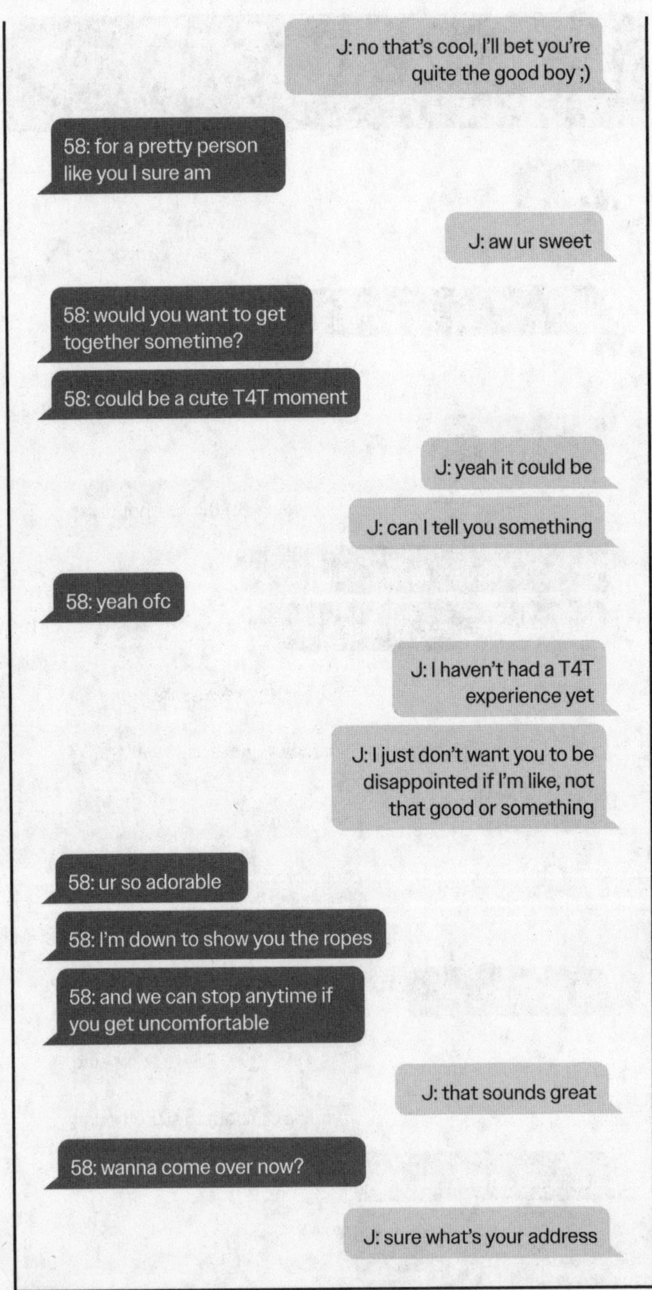
J: no that's cool, I'll bet you're quite the good boy ;)
58: for a pretty person like you I sure am
J: aw ur sweet
58: would you want to get together sometime?
58: could be a cute T4T moment
J: yeah it could be
J: can I tell you something
58: yeah ofc
J: I haven't had a T4T experience yet
J: I just don't want you to be disappointed if I'm like, not that good or something
58: ur so adorable
58: I'm down to show you the ropes
58: and we can stop anytime if you get uncomfortable
J: that sounds great
58: wanna come over now?
J: sure what's your address

I make it halfway down the block to where my Lyft will be waiting. My teeth chatter, though it was at least seventy-five degrees. I had changed my underwear too many times: jockstrap to brief to sheer brief back to jockstrap and settling on the second pair of briefs. None of them were sexy or femme enough. I check my phone. *Four Minutes Away!* I check his profile. Still cute. I scroll through our chat, realizing we hadn't exchanged a single nude. I can't remember the last time a guy invited me over without first thoroughly inspecting multiple digital images of my asshole.

Maybe he actually likes me for me, I think, then rolled my eyes for thinking it. I focus my mind on what is about to happen: kissing this boy with his newly grown mustache, asking if I can run my hands down his binder or if that was off-limits, letting him suck my dick, telling him he's a good boy. I think of him fixing a strap on, climbing on top of me, and I think of asking him to stop. Just to test him, to see if he meant what he said about stopping at the Rape or Not Rape crossroads. In my mind, he will stop, he will dismount, we will lie there, and talk. He will not ask me to leave, he will ask me thoughtful questions and show me silly videos on YouTube and I will maybe kiss his shoulder.

Two Minutes Away!

I want to cry. I nearly start. In a frenzy I cancel the Lyft, and message him.

J: sorry, something came up and
I can't tonight.

I try not to think of his disappointment. I think about the cracks in the sidewalk and the frayed hem of my T-shirt and my sleeping grandfather and literally anything else. I tell myself I did the right thing. I tell myself to stop crying on the street like a child. I tell myself this is for the better. I stuff my hands in my pockets and grit my teeth to quell the overwhelming thought that keeps coming: He probably wouldn't like me anyway.

Finn, Before

Sunday morning split the blinds with sunshine. New York City car horns sparked at my ears. A soft snore harmonized with the air conditioner. I couldn't bring myself to open my eyes; either Finn would be there, and I'd have a few blissful moments under the comforter with him before he ran off to wherever he had to go, or it was all a dream, and I'd be faced with my pillow and a pit in my stomach.

I peeked. Blond hair brushed my eyelashes. Warmth thumped under our palms. We had fallen asleep holding hands. Gross. Divine.

He must've felt me wake because in one tectonic shift, eyes still closed, he slid his arm under my pillow, wriggled his legs around mine, and landed his head on my chest. If there were car horns or air conditioners or sunlight I didn't notice.

A long pause.

"I can feel your heartbeat."

"You are suuuuch a faggot, oh my god," I murmured, though I'm sure he felt my heart's pace quicken.

"It's so fast!"

"It always is," I assured him.

He paused. "I like your heart."

"Hey." I poked at his Abercrombie shoulder.

"Hey!" he whined. I picked his head up and rolled it over so I could see into his matching oceans.

"I like your heart too."

It had only been three weeks. It felt serious to say this, or perhaps it was special because I'd never said to anyone the words *I like your heart* before. It's a nice warm-up for saying all the bigger things we hadn't yet: I want to keep seeing you, I want to be with you, will you be my boyfriend, I love you.

"Shut upppp," he mumbled and kissed my chin. "Can I kiss you?"

"But morning brea—"

"I don't care."

Another tectonic shift, his plates landing squarely on mine, a kiss like lava. I thought I'd melt into the pillows, a river of creamy wax, nothing left but the twitching wick of a heartbeat that rapped against his chest.

"It's still so fast," he said, platinum strands hovering over my eyebrows.

"It's because I'm nervous! I'm still not used to this!"

"Well, get used to it."

"Sure, sure, I'll get right on that."

I was suddenly aware of my eye crust and my cowlick and the sticky skin on my back from sweating against a boy in the July summer, and I heard myself say, "Are you used to this?"

He stopped. I was serious. He considered. "No, not exactly."

"Tell me more."

"Do you want the truth?"

Beat beat beatbeatbeatbeat. "Always."

He sat up, kneading the comforter at his belly button. "Honestly? It's been a long time since I've dated anyone. Not that we've said we're dating or anything, but I guess maybe we are? I just—after my ex, I decided I wanted to be alone and, you know, have my slut phase or whatever and not get tied up into anything, especially considering this job is going to take me to the other side of the world . . . but I can't seem to stay away from you, and I guess that's, well, scary."

I wasn't sure where to start, what to respond to. "Thank you for sharing that."

He shrugged.

"No, I mean it." I swallowed. "I really didn't know where your head was, and I've been wondering but I didn't want to put any pressure on you. Plus, I was kinda embarrassed about the other night—"

"The crying?"

"Yes, the crying, thank you for the reminder! Look, I don't want you to jump into anything you're not ready for. I . . . I really like being with you and I want to see where that goes. It feels like we're dating and it's scary for me to say but I want to be dating you. Or at least starting to. We don't need to put labels or anything yet and I'm not trying to cockblock your slut phase but . . . that's where my head is."

He looked up, and then back at me with a huff. "I hate these conversations."

I had fucked up. *Great*. "Why?"

"Because we sound like a cheesy rom-com, and that is for sure not my vibe."

"I think it is your vibe," I teased. "You started it."

His jaw slackened, a protest.

"Don't give me that look! You started this!"

"And as it turns out I liked it, because now I know that you want to date me."

My turn for the jaw. "Of course I want to date you!"

"Oh yeah?"

"Um, yeah! Were you questioning that?"

"It doesn't matter now," he said, removing the strategically placed comforter. I kicked the rest of my sheets off in response.

"So, are we like, together?"

He crawled toward me. Another tectonic shift, a river of lava, a puddle of wax. I wanted him, I wanted him, I wanted him.

"Yeah," he breathed. "We're together."

The arrow landed. I had him, I had him, I had him.

The oven light clock informs me we're preparing dinner at 4:06 p.m., but if it said 11:06 my body would have believed it. My grandfather, despite the dementia, remains an early riser, keeping us on our toes. Breakfast, puzzles, *The Andy Griffith Show* reruns, repeat, hope he doesn't remember this one, hope we don't go mad. My grandmother is taking a nap. I have pulled the green beans from the second drawer of the refrigerator. We handpicked them from the farmer's market last Sunday because if he is going to die, he will die having eaten fresh food. We say we are doing it for him, but really it's our excuse to keep ourselves eating. If grief doesn't pull the appetite, the anxiety about it will scrape your stomach clean.

I let four eggs thunk into an open pot of boiling water, then immediately regret the thunking as one bursts with a mushroom cloud of yellow. I enlist a ladle to fish out the egg and its yellow cloud, slingshotting it across the kitchen into the sink disposal.

"Whoa, there!" My grandfather, wide-eyed, begins clapping. "Atta boy!"

My toss was good. He is laughing. I am the local sports phenom of the kitchen.

"Would you like to help me with dinner?" According to the experts at our local Memory Center it is important to involve Alzheimer's patients in routine, daily tasks while they can still handle them, as it offers them a sense of belonging and purpose. I pretend that doesn't sound like a page out of a book entitled something akin to *How to Raise Emotionally Competent Children in the Modern Age* and await his response.

"Well, yes!" He nods and pushes his joystick forward. He curves around the counter and settles at the family dining room table—oak wood, an heirloom from my great-grandfather. To preserve its finish, I slide a cutting board in front of him topped with a heap of raw green beans.

"Will you cut the tips off of these for me so I can steam them for dinner?"

"Where is my wife?"

"She's coming, she's just taking a nap."

"Oh, oh."

I restart. "Will you cut the tips off of these for me so I can steam them for dinner?"

"Well, absolutely!"

He plucks a singular bean from the heap and sets it in the center of his cutting board. I offer him a paring knife—blade toward me—which he accepts. He looks at it for half a second too long, and then proceeds to the task with the dull side. He studies the green bean (unmoored, tips intact) and then the knife. My hand reaches for the knife—this was a poor idea after all, I should have him watch *Andy Griffith* or let him hand me the beans or something else—when he flips the knife over and slices with alacrity.

"There!" He places the beheaded legume in the pot for steaming and pulls another from the heap.

"Thought this knife didn't work for a minute there." He cuts, cuts, deposits. "Imagine that?"

Imagine that.

Do you think the 9/11 memorial is a bottom?

Or am I being position-ist because it has a huge, gaping hole

The last time I had a huge gaping hole I was definitely a bottom so I'm just synthesizing here

The only way to test this hypothesis is if you bring a bunch of tops to the 9/11 memorial and see if they get hard but the problem is I never seem to date them long enough to bring them to this special place

Another issue I'm flagging here is that if they got hard how would I know whether that had to do with the 9/11 memorial or these four-inch-inseam jean shorts I thrifted

This is what we call a "confounding variable" in science.

Also, if they did get hard how could we say (with statistical significance) that they aren't turned on by the trauma of it all because guys who get hard at trauma are pretty likely to be rapists, I'd say

The 9/11-memorial-is-a-bottom theory kinda makes sense because (and I'm assuming here) Osama was a top

I know this because technically straight men are tops. At least, a lot of them are? I guess??

I suppose I should employ my own politic and not assume someone's sexuality but recall page 50, many wives, ten-year-old daughter (lest we forget)

And in order to have many wives and children you have to top . . . technically

I can entertain the idea that Osama bin Laden was a Vers Bicon later but I am really not ready for intercommunity blowback from bisexuals right now so you will have to wait for another time to get riled up over this

Back to the point: Tops tend to have destructive tendencies (speaking from personal experience) and I'd say Osama had destructive tendencies at the very least

Another distinguishing feature of tops is that they penetrate (obvious, you knew this) and I'd say that's what Osama did to the towers

Actually wait Osama didn't fly any of the planes . . . does that make him a passive top instead? Or were all the guys who hijacked the planes also bottoms because they listened to him like good little boys?

This must be what gays on Twitter mean when they say "Bottom on bottom crime"

There is something romantic about all of this (tenderness of men listening to each other's feelings?) but I'll let you sort that out for yourselves

The whole situation is very Montagues/Capulets when you think of the whole U.S. vs. Middle East, people with power fighting, penetration leading to the ultimate demise, etc.

There's another case for the 9/11 memorial not being a bottom, but someone with a vagina because it self-lubricates

I understand this self-lubrication theory could be problematic, I'm just thinking out loud

Not all of us can self-lubricate, sometimes we just cry, and that's the wrong orifice

(The 9/11 memorial does not seem to have this problem but I do)

This is why I have a recurring supply of Gun Oil!

No fewer than nine of you had to look up Gun Oil and learned I was not plotting war crimes I was referencing a slick brand of premium lubricant of which the 9/11 memorial does not need because, as I mentioned, it self-lubricates

However!!! Vagina owners also often use lube (or might want to!) because sometimes you need a little extra

Like how we all need "a little extra" security in TSA after 9/11 so government officials can harass Brown people and racially profile everyone else, this concept is totally working and not harmful at all and absolutely worth getting to the airport two hours before my plane takes off, which makes a two-hour flight like a seven-hour travel day UGHHHH the racism of it all

Osama also needed "a little extra" but it wasn't Gun Oil it was actual guns or, as Dick Cheney famously said, "weapons of mass destruction"

Finnegan was also a top; are you seeing the similarities?

He claimed to be vers but that never happened

How many of Osama's wives were told the same story? We should start a support group

Speaking of vers remember when they said they could reverse the planes? That did not happen

There is a conspiracy theory that the plane headed for the Capitol building was shot down by the U.S. military because that was the safer option for everyone in the Capitol/D.C. Metro area

I think about this with rapists a lot because how do we target them and shoot them down before they attack other people??

I'm not saying they deserve to die (maybe they do); I'm saying it would be nice to have a radar that beeps so you know you're about to collide with one on Grindr on a midnight in October despite the fact that he's super hot and says nice things about you and you miss Finnegan but you go over anyway—

Gun Oil!!!!

How much lubricant is aboard submarines, does anyone know?

And if there's a lot how much of it is Swiss Navy?

GET IT

Wait one more—if it is Swiss Navy is it ~water based~????

(Ok, I'm done)

A List of Things You Can Find in an Article About 9/11 That I've Also Said in Bed:

- Obliterate
- Fuck
- That was hot
- This is on fire
- I'm falling
- Oh shit another one
- Are you sure this is ok?
- Can you see out the window
- I can't breathe
- It's coming
- I'm coming
- Again?
- Hey, are you ok?

Approximately 3,000 people died in 9/11; how many of them do you think were sex offenders?

> Make that 3,001 since we should probably count my inner child

And if they were sex offenders does that undercut our empathy for their deaths?

> Imagine if, say, Mr. Anderson was on that plane. I would probably have not been molested and if given the choice I'd go with tragic-death-by-hijacking over showing a seven-year-old your nuts on school property and saying, "You can touch them if you want."
>
> > "If you want" is the part that really gets me. As IF you can somehow manufacture consent for a seven-year-old you're literally molesting???? Like fuck OFF the illusion of choice, even the mere implication I had one is beyond vile

You gotta wonder if anyone has been molested on a plane

Probably hard to do, those bathrooms are notoriously small and people don't usually leave their kids unattended for fear they'll be kidnapped or impounded or whatever

My proofreader has informed me there was a highly publicized case about this in 2023. I read the article; he circumvented the small bathroom issue by waiting until the cabin lights dimmed and molesting her right there in the seat

Pedophiles are getting so advanced these days, they don't even need the back closet of the music room or a tiny bathroom; they just need you to fall asleep on a red-eye

Yikes, that's dark

Just like the final moments of Mr. Anderson's life if he'd take a flight out of Boston Logan that morning

Imagine you're trying to join the mile-high club with your consenting adult partner and you overhear your plane literally getting hijacked by al-Qaeda

I probably wouldn't have heard this because I would've been in ecstasy and if I'm gonna go down with the hijacking I wanna do it with someone going down on me

Hijacking? More like jack-you-off-in-the-lavatory-because-we're-all-gonna-die-anyway, Steven

I don't know a Steven, but if you knew a Steven on those planes I'm genuinely so sorry

I would've traded him for Mr. Anderson

I bet you would've too

This is what we call a "confounding variable" in life.

Finn, Before

The stressful part wasn't actually the party, it was that at this particular party I was meeting all of his friends. I was subletting in the West Village, where old money manifested as a walk-in closet and more than one bathroom for the unit. His friends were meeting us there. I'm not much for hosting but I was one for making Finn happy, and besides, when would I have an apartment this nice to show off again?

The thrum of bodies in space in this apartment should've been sweatier—it was summer—but somehow the warmth was pleasing. Thigh Tattoo arrived first, donning cutoff jean shorts exposing the art that became his namesake. Well, mental namesake. (Note: "art" is a generous term here; I would hardly call a blue-and-red dragon that bubbled over one's quadricep at a forty-five-degree angle "high art," but alas I didn't get it inked on my body so beauty is in the eye of the beholder or whatever they say.) He kissed Finn on the cheek and shot me a look out of the corner of his eye.

"He was mine first you little twit-sack, watch the fuck out."

Ok, he didn't actually say that, but he might as well have. And I don't really know why I threw in "twit-sack"; it just sounded like something he would say? He kicked his basic, white sneakers by the door. I offered a smile. You get the point.

Redhead from Childhood was next, who naturally brought three other people I didn't know, but who flung her arms around me the moment I opened the door so I had no time to question.

"I'VEHEARDSOMUCHABOUTYOU!!!!" she said louder than anyone expected. "Oh my goodness, Finny??? They are BEAUTIFUL." She petted my coif the way one smooths the head of a neighbor's house cat and thunked a bottle of wine into my sternum.

"Oh, sorry love!" I wondered where the accent came from and how she'd ended up neighbors with "Finny" when they were six, but the impact to my skin interrupted my thoughts.

"Hope this is alright, 's'all I've got!" she said, uncoiling a lock of hair from her spaghetti strap. "You fancy a good rosé, don't you?"

"Oh, well my last name is Rose, so it's kind of—"

"PERFECT!!" she screeched and did a bounce in place before plunging her way toward Thigh Tattoo. "You right bitch, how ARE you?" She trailed off and I turned to Finn.

He put his arm around my shoulders and kissed my temple. "She's always like that." Another kiss, longer. "Don't worry, she already loves you, they all will."

I suppose he was right. One by one (or six at a time, in one case) they piled in—college friends, boyfriends of college friends, that one girl from the last show he did, her cousin who she was staying with and was it ok that she brought her? A mosaic of ponytails and Fjällräven bags and nonnormative pronouns. For some reason I had worn a polo shirt, which, come to think of it, probably made me look silly.

They all seemed to know me—Septum Piercing #2 and her boyfriend heard about the last show I did because Finn told them. Four of his classmates had seen my musical theater videos on YouTube because Finn sent them, and even Thigh Tattoo said the place was nice and he heard I could sing. Redhead from Childhood was sweet, she corrected a stray boyfriend when he misgendered me before his girlfriend (college classmate?) could scold him.

Beers peppered the main table and three blonde girls talking about Sutton Foster had commandeered the rosé. I perched on the arm of the couch next to Finn, who was laughing with Thigh Tattoo about some prank they pulled on one of the Sutton girls sophomore year. Fistfuls of chips found their way to people's mouths, the inevitable who-is-your-favorite-Elphaba debate rallied us around the TV. I had mostly been quiet, but eventually found myself fiercely defending Ana Gasteyer's "The Wizard and I" to an uproarious crowd, clicker in hand, now sweating through my polo in the summer heat. I didn't care, they were listening, they were laughing, they liked me, which meant Finn would be happy. Belonging starts somewhere.

At some point during the *SNL* Sketch YouTube Tour of the night, I slunk down from my arm into the couch next to Finn, who looked over and immediately pulled me in.

"Hi, baby," he said while the room was distracted with Maya Rudolph.

I kissed him. "Hi right back."

He smiled and the room around me faded. Maya went near silent in the background, and I whispered, "Do you think they like me?"

He rolled his eyes and squeezed the back of my neck with the crook of his elbow. "Of course they do, babe. What's not to like?"

I let my head fall onto his shoulder, he brushed my arm with his thumb. At some point I must've fallen asleep—the rosé, the affirmation, the job-well-done, the adrenaline release all tugging my eyelids shut.

I don't know how long he let me stay asleep on his shoulder amidst all his friends, but the next thing I remember my sleeping head was lolling against his chest, and he was carrying me through the doorway, into my bedroom. He slid me under the comforter and switched the AC unit on. It hummed like my heartbeat. He bent down and ran his fingers through my wilted coif the way someone pets their childhood cat.

"She's right," he whispered. "You really are beautiful."

He turned off the light, and I could hear the thrum of bodies beyond the door that had clearly found the karaoke machine. Their laughter welcomed him back into the room. A mere two weeks later when he left for work on the other side of the world I would lie in my bed, willing myself to remember the pitch of their laughter, how many of them were still there, how soft the door clicked when he left.

I hope death is like that.

I hope death feels like your lover carrying you to bed in the middle of the party.

I hope, at my Funeral Pregame, someone slips me into the next room while everyone is distracted with board games or karaoke or beltress compilations.

I hope that's how I go.

I hope I can hear the laughter from the next room.

"James?" My grandmother's hushed whisper sails through the midnight kitchen like a dart.

"Yes?" I was still up for some reason or other.

"I think it's time . . ."

I leapt to my feet, socks pattering across the hardwood floor. "Should we call someone?"

"No, let's . . . let's just listen." She adjusts her flannel, and we cross into the bedroom.

My grandfather is sleeping almost soundlessly. He has not left this bed in three days, which is unusual. We had anticipated this would mark the next stage of the disease, but we had not anticipated him to pass so soon.

I stood next to her, unsure what to do. Should we watch? Is it appropriate to watch someone die? Should we each take one of his hands? Would that startle him? A snore tickled at the back of his throat, distracting me from my thought process. Another snore, this one louder.

"Well, maybe not . . ." My grandmother glanced at me. "I thought it sounded like the death rattle but maybe . . ."

"Maybe he was just snoring?"

"Maybe he was just snoring!"

We tried to laugh in whispers, but failed. We scurried into the bathroom and shut the door, giggling ourselves into delirium. He wasn't dying, he was just snoring. And we were laughing. What a relief. My grandmother clutched against the ADA bar next to the toilet while I doubled over the countertop. I willed the notes escaping my lips to burrow into the fissures in the tile, where the cement might hold the joy tight in its bubbles, releasing it when we would again need it most.

Texts I Wish Finn Would Still Send Me:

1. I really love what you said about challenging weight loss goals as fatphobic it's giving me a lot to think about

2. I may be drnkk by god i miss you

3. Had a cute thought about u on da bus comin home 2nite
4. I ve said for a long time i need someone who will call me on my bullshit but not be a dick about it or try to change me and I feel like you do that

5. I miss u. Bummer.

6. Ugh ur so sweet

7. Staaaaahp ur the cutest

8. Hoenstly felt so shitty this week can i call u for 5 minutes

9. Are u KIDDING ME
10. Like are you for fucking JOKES
11. I'm making that pic my lockscreen

12. You got this baby

13. What are u doin Saturday

14. Oh lol i thought you got the tickets

15. Running 4 minutes late

16. No i'm stuck on the B train

17. Remind me your favorite color

18. GOOD MORNING

19. I got a lil bummed
20. Bc when i miss ppl i look at the moon to miss them less
21. Bc we're looking at the same moon and that comforts me
22. [moon pic]
23. But we ain't lookin at the same moon

24. I've been staring at my phone under your messages trying to figure out what to say to you. I knew I wanted to say something I just couldn't figure out what
25. You're amazing
26. And I adore spending time with you
27. And I don't know what else to say other than that. But you have me truly speechless.

28. Just took the myers Briggs bc i'm STILL awake
29. I got ENFP and I'm shiggity shaggy shook

30. Wow legit can't sleep bc I'm thinking about snuggling you this is gr8
31. Me again, I got to sleep, prob had dreams about you but idk bc I rarely remember my drea,s and woke up a few minutes ago thinking about you and now I can't get back to sleep. I wish i could see you tomorowwwww
32. Or today. You know what i mean.

33. Ur voice is pretty

34. Still thinking ab kissin u

35. hi

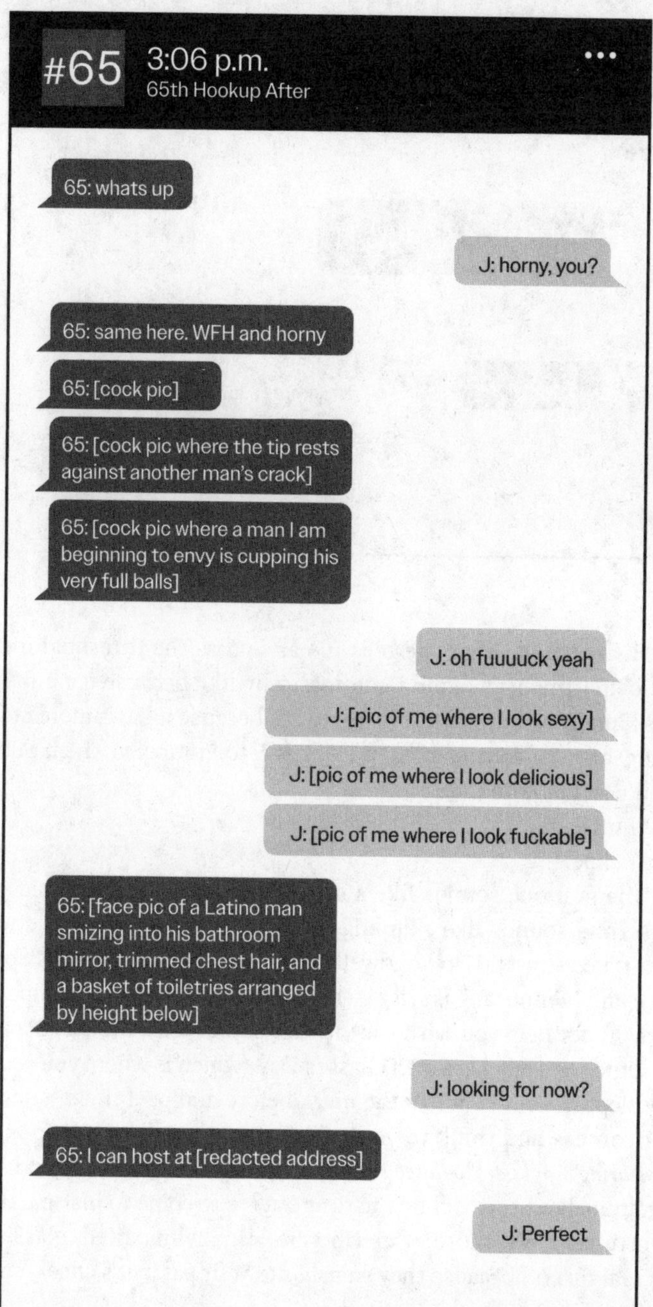
#65
3:06 p.m.
65th Hookup After
65: whats up
J: horny, you?
65: same here. WFH and horny
65: [cock pic]
65: [cock pic where the tip rests against another man's crack]
65: [cock pic where a man I am beginning to envy is cupping his very full balls]
J: oh fuuuuck yeah
J: [pic of me where I look sexy]
J: [pic of me where I look delicious]
J: [pic of me where I look fuckable]
65: [face pic of a Latino man smizing into his bathroom mirror, trimmed chest hair, and a basket of toiletries arranged by height below]
J: looking for now?
65: I can host at [redacted address]
J: Perfect

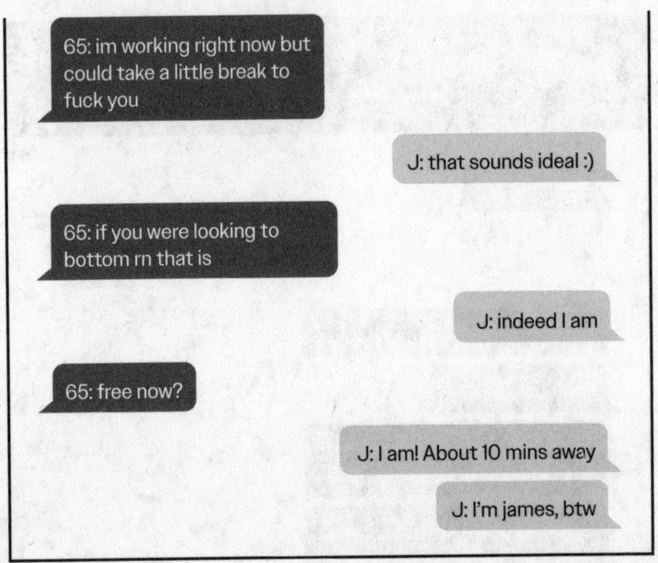

His name is Felipé, he tells me as I cross the threshold into his studio apartment, a name I automatically like because it's a fricative like "Finnegan" but way more fun to say because it has a more creative arrangement of consonants, and a clear *E* to *I* ratio. Say them out loud if you don't believe me.

"Finnegan."

"Felipé."

The first one sounds like a sunk rock in an algae-infested pond, the second sounds like skipping rocks in a teen beach movie with a sepia-toned sunset. (Do not dwell on the fact that "Felipé" is a Spanish name and "Finnegan" is Irish, which means they are not comparable; that will not help you with the visuals. Sunk rocks. Stones. Sepia.)

Unfortunately I am on a Glasses Day (which is where you accidentally slept in your contacts the night before and peel them, sticky, off your corneas and think to yourself, *fuck me, how did this happen, guess I'm wearing my glasses today so I don't ruin my sight at twenty-six*) and I have forgotten about this fact by the time I agree to come to his apartment. Unfortunately for those of us who are visually impaired, glasses can be a real turnoff because they smash into your partner's cheek/crotch/

hole/vagina, and they fog up and you're always afraid you're going to break them if the sex veers aerobic and so it's best to remove them despite the fact that you rob yourself of the joy of seeing your partner utterly enraptured with you and your sexy aerobic self. No matter! Carpe diem! Maybe he'll be uglier than his photos and I'll want to take off my glasses and imagine someone else.

In fact, I'm half-correct, he doesn't really look like his photo. We tumble out of our clothes and through the routine (*hey/how are you/ thanks for coming/can I put my shoes here?*) and all the while I'm wondering how someone's curls can ornament their eyebrows with such regality. Or why the baritone of his voice warms my chest like a chocolate mocha with two pumps of caramel in December. Suddenly I'm wishing I could be the ink that runs vertical from armpit to hip bone. Or the music notes tattoo shelved on his clavicle. Or the constellation etched into his back right shoulder revealed to me as he pulls a towel over the bed. Orion's belt glistens—I've never seen that shade of yellow ink on skin before. Maybe everything that touched him became prettier.

With this thought I touch his bicep and he pulls me in for a kiss.

"Thanks for coming over, cutie."

"You already said that." I giggle.

I run my hands up the vertical tattoo and kiss the melody on his collar bone. He works my neck, moving my hair out of his tongue's way with the backside of his fingers. I silently curse myself for not bringing a hair tie. His fade is so sleek, the crown of curls intact. My untamable mane sprawls past my shoulders like a fistful of cooked spaghetti whacked against a countertop. I feel silly for liking him.

"Mmm." He returns to my lips, and I feel the evidence of the blood rush between his legs.

I grin. "Ok, wow."

"You want it?"

I rediscover (to my horror!) I am wearing my glasses, partially because his nose knocks against them and partially because I want to blow him and realize they'd be in the way. If I keep them on for the blowjob they'll fog up and restrict my neck mobility; if I take them off, I won't be able to see how much he's enjoying (or worse, tolerating) my work.

"I can't believe I'm wearing these, oh my god."

He says nothing.

"I usually wear contacts," I clarify.

"I see." Undeterred, he uses the next six kisses to pull me onto the bed. His thighs drip over his legs, which fold underneath him. His penis bobs up at me. It's cruel to leave a dick like that unsucked.

Fuck it. I set my glasses on his bedside table, swing the spaghetti over one shoulder, and get to work. Before long I hear the words "flip over, baby," coated in waxy baritone. I flip over, baby.

What you need to understand before we proceed is how many tops are resistant to rimming. I know, you'd think the subset of gay men who repeatedly goon off to ass pics would be more inclined to eat a girl out, but alas we are sixty-something men into this adventure and how many of them gave me the rimjob I deserved? Maybe four?

(There is more to say about the inequalities of the blowjob-to-rimjob ratio in queer communities, and I will write some essay of cultural criticism about this eventually but for now you'll have to settle for a preview because I need to finish creating this art piece.)

My theory of oral sex inequality is that rimming doesn't give tops as much pleasure so they aren't as inclined to do it. Bottoms give blowjobs, on the other hand, because they're a tool of submission—it can be quite fun when a hunk twice your size says he wants to "fuck your throat like a pussy" right before following through on his word. Being a good little mouth hole gets some of us off because we are, indeed, getting a dick inside of us. (Woohoo! Score!)

Rimjobs? More complicated. You have to get your bottom in precisely the right position, and there's a lot to consider. Angle, hole placement, cheek thickness, how clean is it actually? How the hole puckers, your neck flexibility, elbow-to-cheek-to-pillow ratio (Pythagorean if you really think about it), how long your tongue is, and how dexterous. It can really make or break the experience, let me tell you. Sucking dick? Any position, any way, men just wanna get their dick wet and as long as you're providing the wetness it'll work.*

---

*Some top is going to read this and have a guttural reaction, nay even be insulted, because he takes his rimjob work quite seriously and doesn't believe it's as complicated as I say. He has spent years perfecting his craft, writing op-eds on "bottomphobia," and is taking up the mantle of righting the cultural wrong of un-rimmed-yet-still-fucked bottoms. I welcome him to contact me directly at topsfrompage90@gmail.com, thank you so much.

ALL OF THIS TO SAY, when a guy is working from home and says, "I can take a little break to fuck you," rarely—if ever—does that mean he's going to ask you to sit on his face while he tongues you six ways to Sunday.

Not Felipé! This man slides his vertical tattooed self underneath me, takes one hand to each ass cheek, and goes for it as if he invented anilingus. This man writes love letters with his tongue. In cursive. It's as if he's digging his way to the other side of the world and the entry point is my (and I quote) "tight little hole." I try to return the favor by continuing to suck the dick that is in front of me, but one devastatingly good lick later I unintentionally collapse on his chest with his cock jammed down my trachea. He moans so deep my liver vibrates.

It's as if he's saying, "Get the Finnegan out of here, it's Felipé's turn."

Oh, it certainly is his turn.

As we all know, I find doggy a notoriously difficult position. This is probably because of what Finnegan once said about how he puts guys in doggy when he "doesn't want to look at them anymore" and that imprinted on the side of my brain that houses "Insecurities" and "Post-Traumatic Stress Disorder." It's also rather . . . hard to take a dick that way! Again, some of you may disagree, and maybe some of your holes are just better placed or your lumbar spines have more give, but I simply cannot spend any time on all fours without significant warm-up. I also cannot have sex without lube, because unlike our good friend the 9/11 memorial, I do not self-lubricate.

So, if I told you that a man fucked me in doggy with no lube, I would need you to be HORRIFIED. Unless that man was Felipé. Because once he's installed a brand-new plumbing system inside me with his tongue he sets me on all fours and whispers in my ear, "Are you ready, babe?"

I nod vigorously. He slides in without so much as a wince from me. Remember that part about not self-lubricating? I don't know what is going on today, but I am giving the 9/11 memorial stiff competition for Gushiest Hole.* Remember how I said I couldn't do doggy because my lumbar is too stiff? For Felipé I'm a horseshoe.

---

*Please always use lube! You can really hurt yourself or your partner without it. Do NOT romanticize lubeless sex, do as I say, not as I did with Felipé. You are not the 9/11 memorial; you are a person.

This man thrusts me into a mental orbit that can only be described as the dicking down of a lifetime, and right as he is about to cum he puts his arm around my chest and kisses my lips from behind. Baritone moans shoot down my tongue while he shoots inside me. I will not even subject you to my woes of the rarities of a man going through the neck-craning effort to kiss you while he's hitting it from the back, let alone while he cums. So many tops won't even look at you when they cum, let alone allow you to share the moment mouth-to-mouth with a hand around your throat. Love, I now know, looks like this.

Then, after we collapse, it starts. I know what you're thinking (dammit, James, don't cry!) and I didn't!!! I felt leakage. The kind of leakage when his little swimmies are going the wrong direction in your colon and threatening to plop onto his comforter.

"I'll be right back," I say, clenched and crawling off the bed. I fumble my glasses back over my ears and scurry to the bathroom, phone in hand. I let the sink water run so he won't hear me let out a stream of swimmies. I exhale. I reach for a towel to wipe my brow (doggy is hard, remember?), and I see them: two matching white towels with calligraphy "his" and "theirs."

My heart falls into my stomach, pushing the next swimmy stream into the bowl below.

His.

Theirs.

This is a studio apartment. There are only three possible explanations:

1. He uses he/they pronouns and someone got him these expensive-looking monogrammed towels to commemorate his coming out as some form of gender expansive.
2. They were an early wedding gift for me or a hint that he wanted me to be his partner forever, which seems unlikely given that we messaged for the first time less than an hour ago but not completely out of the realm of possibility! Maybe he was trying to earn ally points ahead of time.
3. He uses he/him pronouns and he has a nonbinary partner who uses they/them and they live together and the partner gets anilinguified every night and then the two of them walk

to the shower together after bed-rocking, aerobic sex and Felipé wraps his femme partner and their tame hair and 20/20 vision in a fluffy, gender-affirming towel and says, "You're so beautiful baby, I'm so lucky to be in love with you."

I open my phone to Felipé's profile and scroll:

Pronouns: he/him

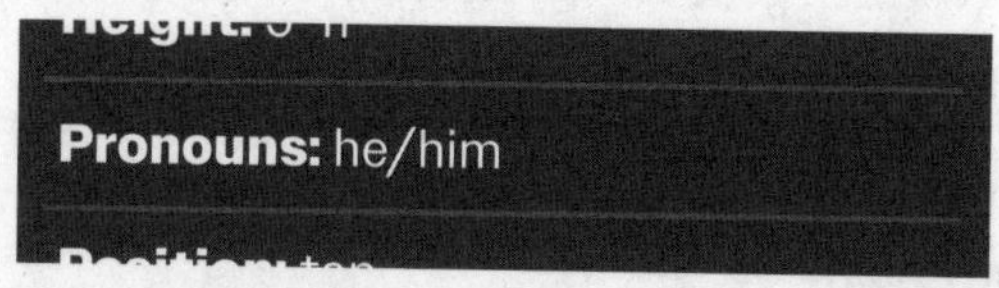

Ok, that takes out Possibility #1. I scroll again, slower.

Relationship Status:
Partnered. Live together, only host when they're out of town.

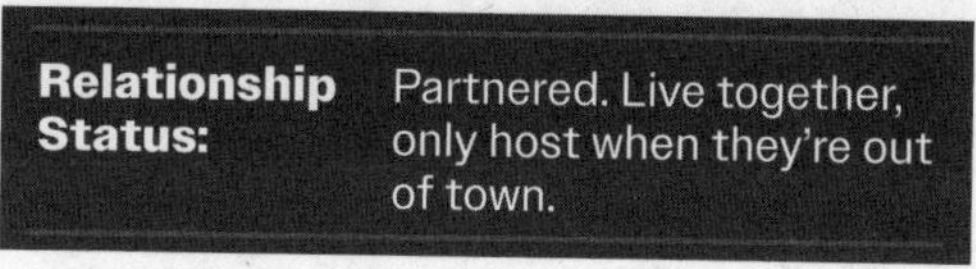

Spaghetti strands hover above my phone. Fuck. He has a nonbinary partner, which means three more things:

1. If a man like Felipé could love a nonbinary person, that meant we were actually lovable.
2. If a man like Felipé was so dedicated to nonbinary pleasure, that meant maybe we deserved to feel it.
3. And if he loved and pleasured someone else, this was the end of the road for us. I didn't want to compete with the towel owner. I didn't want to think about what Felipé's enthusiasm for my pleasure meant about the other sixty-something men from before. I didn't want to see another man and be utterly disappointed by his incompetence with his tongue and with simple parts of speech.

I sit on the toilet, water still running. I feel them coming: the tears, scalding and feverish on my cheeks. I don't move. I let them fall between my legs into the bowl below me and I just . . . feel the pain. My asshole throbs, raw from my lubeless decisions. My heart throbs, embarrassed I got my hopes up when all the information I needed was on a public-facing profile. My eyes puff underneath my glasses. I shift on the toilet. I'm afraid to leave the bathroom. I feel so ugly. Unlike Orion's belt, when I touched him I did not become prettier. My glasses slide down my nose on a flume of tears.

Anxious I'd been gone for too long, I grab the closer towel—*His*—and blot my face. I spin the toilet paper roll in preparation, and then at the last minute I grab *Theirs* and wipe my ass clean. It emerges with a stain clear through the calligraphy.

I instantly regret it.

He is never going to love me.

I regret everything.

I hear it happen: His wheelchair knocks into the lowest cabinet of dining room dishes. The problem isn't the bump, the problem is the time: 1:53 a.m. He has been in bed since 8:30. He is not able to get up on his own. Something has happened.

The pads of my feet make small thumping noises as I run down the staircase and through possible scenarios:

- He had an accident and my grandmother put him in his wheelchair to change the sheets.
- He woke up, restless and agitated, and my grandmother lost that battle and put him in his wheelchair.
- He has somehow gotten strong enough to hoist himself out of bed and slide into his wheelchair alone—a feat he's never accomplished before—and we are oh so fucked.

I am wrong on all three counts. The dining room remains intact. The lowest cabinet of dishes untouched. His wheelchair charges at the port next to the piano. I turn around, looking for further evidence; I find nothing.

The dining room connects to the ADA corridor that leads to my grandparents' room, meaning any lights I turn on would flood their doorless bedroom and wake them. I decide against flipping the switch and continue my investigation in the kitchen. There it is: the steel mixing bowl I used for mashed potatoes this afternoon, belly down on the wood floor. Hours ago, I had placed it haphazardly atop two other bowls to dry on the dish towel. I rinse it, relieved, and place it on a towel of its own this time.

In the darkness I turn to retrace my steps to find I'm not in my grandparents' house at all. I'm walking out of my rapist's room at 1:58 a.m. and down the dark corridor toward what I think is the exit, the front door, the outside world.

"Down the hall to the right," he says, rolling over in bed to change the song on his laptop as if this was routine. My sweatshirt and my scarf are still bunched in my hands. My shoes hang on the hooks of my fingers. Feeling evades my body.

I stop. I hear him breathing. I am barely ten paces from his door. Could he already be asleep? Was he passed out, weary from taking what wasn't his, satisfied with getting what he wanted? Do rapists sleep through the night? The hum of his breath closes in like a swarm of buzzards, their wings as strong as hurricane winds and moist like clouds about to burst. I look to my right. Down the ADA corridor is my grandparents' humidifier guarding the entrance to their room.

I shudder and wipe the sweat from my hairline. I feel the cool wood beneath my feet. I feel the washcloth at my neck. I feel the cup of water at my lips. I wake up hours later to my grandmother asking if everything is alright, telling me it's 6:00 a.m. but I can go back to sleep. When she asks me why I'm sleeping on the couch downstairs I don't have an answer.

Finn, Before

A Scene from a Long-Distance Relationship:

Lights up on JAMES (nonbinary, beautiful, twenty-two) making chocolate chip pancakes. Their phone is propped against the egg carton. Their partner, FINNEGAN (blond, Abercrombie shoulders, twenty-two) calls them on FaceTime from halfway across the world, where he is currently working. This is important because they can only talk mornings and nights with the twelve-hour time difference. It's JAMES's morning, FINN's night.

*** Note from the playwright: While this did happen to the real James and Finnegan, for the purposes of the medium it may be helpful to envision the roles played by various Hollywood actors. For FINN consider Leonardo DiCaprio or Ryan Gosling, for JAMES either Cate Blanchett, Anne Hathaway, or Jessica Chastain. They are all very similar to real-life JAMES in looks, acting chops, and maybe career if they can manage to sell the film rights to this book.*

JAMES. *(answering the phone)* Hey babe, what happened last night?

FINN. You look handsome today, I like this tank top!

JAMES. Thank you, not the point. What happened?

FINN. I was at Arnie's.

JAMES. Yeah, but you always answer me even if you're at his place.

FINN. Is it a problem that I was there?

(JAMES flips the second pancake, the chocolate chips settle.)

JAMES. No, it's fine that you were there, the problem is that we had planned to talk but I didn't hear anything from you so I was worried and—

FINN. *(cutting them off with a huff)* You were jealous, weren't you?

JAMES. I don't know if I was jealous so much as worried and kinda confused. I mean, I assumed you were at Arnie's, and I figured that meant you two would probably have sex and that's ok with me—

FINN. James, we talked about this.

JAMES. Finn, I know we talked about this. This isn't about the open relationship, this is about your canceling plans. Ghosting me, essentially.

FINN. I thought we were gonna talk tomorrow.

JAMES. Well we are, this is technically tomorrow for me.

FINN. But not for me, I'm on Japan time.

JAMES. *(sighing)* Ok, you know that's not what I mean though. *(They turn the burner down.)* I felt jilted last night. I had a weird day and I was really looking forward to talking to you. This has been hard, not seeing you, and I'm doing my best to adjust my expectations, but if you don't communicate that a plan has changed then it just, like, sucks when I can't talk to you and I don't know why.

FINN. I hear you. *(Beat.)* I definitely could've communicated better.

JAMES. *(sincerely)* Thank you.

FINN. I was also drunk, and that well, complicated things.

JAMES. Oh, you were drunk?

FINN. Are you judging?

JAMES. I am not! I just didn't know that was the plan for a Wednesday night.

FINN. Just like you didn't know it was the plan to get dicked down by that hung pilot last week in between his delivery shifts—

JAMES. That was a surprise! I didn't plan it, it just happened! *(Beat.)* Oh, look who's jealous now, huh?

FINN. I'm not jealous! I'm glad you had good sex.

JAMES. I wish it was you though. *(They test the pancakes. Not ready yet.)* Do you ever think that, when you're hooking up with Arnie?

FINN. Think what?

JAMES. That you miss me, or that you'd rather be with me? In that moment?

FINN. I've never really thought about it that way. When I'm with you, I'm with you, and when I'm with him it's just . . . sex. It doesn't really mean anything. So

I'm not comparing it to you because it lives in such a different place in my head.

JAMES. I'll take that, it's sweet. *(The first one is ready to be flipped. They slide the spatula underneath and flip flawlessly.)* Well then, while we're on the topic, how was sex with Arnie last night?

FINN. That's actually something I wanted to talk to you about . . .

JAMES. Oh?

FINN. Yeah, this morning when I lef—

JAMES. You slept over?

FINN. Yeah.

JAMES. That's a . . . that's a first, right?

FINN. Are you upset?

JAMES. No, I'm just taking it in.

FINN. Because it's not against the rul—

JAMES. I know, the only rule is condoms with everyone else so we don't have to use them with each other. We didn't say anything about sleepovers because I guess I just . . . hadn't considered it?

FINN. So that's really the thing. *(He shifts uncomfortably. JAMES flips the second pancake.)* This morning when I was leaving I couldn't find the condom.

JAMES. What do you mean?

FINN. Well, like, I always throw it away in the trash can in his bathroom but I didn't see it.

JAMES. I don't follow. What are you saying?

FINN. I'm saying I was drun–

JAMES. You already told me that.

FINN. *(overlapping)* And I don't really rem–

JAMES. Remember where you put the condo–

FINN. No, I'm saying that–

JAMES. Oh, shit. *(Beat.)* You don't think you used one.

FINN. *(hanging his head)* I was drunk, I don't remember putting one on, I don't really remember a lot of it–

JAMES. But Arnie knows about us, right?

(The spatula drips batter on the counter. JAMES doesn't notice.)

FINN. Yeah, he does.

JAMES. So he knows the rules and he would've had you put one on, right?

FINN. Well that's the thing. Last week he asked me if I would ask you if we could have sex without one. He says it doesn't feel the same and–

JAMES. I'm sorry, what? *(They slide the pancakes onto a plate so they won't burn.)* Some guy who doesn't even know me is asking for us to rewrite the agreements of our open relationship so you can fuck him raw? That doesn't sit right with me.

FINN. Babe, I know, I didn't think it would—

JAMES. Why didn't you tell me this?

FINN. James, I don't want to change the rules of our relationship. I like our agreements. I didn't bring it up because I don't want them to change, and I don't really want to fuck him raw.

JAMES. *(leveling)* Ok. So then you did or you didn't use a condom?

FINN. That's what I'm trying to tell you, I don't know. I don't think we did. I checked my backpack this morning and there's still one in there, and I don't remember if I brought two or just one but I'm really afraid we didn't use one.

JAMES. Did you ask him?

FINN. He was drunk too.

JAMES. But did you ask him?

FINN. Yeah, he said he doesn't remember.

JAMES. Of course he would say that.

FINN. What's that supposed to mean?

JAMES. Exactly what I said, of course he would say that. Because if you did use a condom then everything would be fine, but if he casts a tiny shadow of a doubt in your mind then he knows you'll have to tell me and he knows we'll fight about it and who is that great for? Him! Because then he gets a better shot at being with you!

FINN. You sound crazy.

JAMES. Am I wrong, though?

(FINN is silent for a moment. JAMES is holding it together.)

FINN. Baby, please don't do this, I didn't mean t–

JAMES. So basically, what you're saying is . . . you cheated on me.

FINN. *(carefully)* I wouldn't put it that way–

JAMES. How would you put it? Because we had an agreement, and one of us broke it, and it wasn't me.

FINN. Whoa, it was an accident!

JAMES. Oh, you just accidentally put your raw cock inside some guy who has been begging for it for God knows how long?

FINN. I was drunk!

JAMES. But you remember having sex?

FINN. Yes.

JAMES. So you were sober enough to remember having sex, but drunk enough to forget a condom?

FINN. Well, I don't really know if I was sober enough to have sex–

JAMES. Whoa, ok, that's a . . . that's a completely different story. *(Gently now.)* Were you sober enough to consent to this? *(FINN doesn't answer.)* Babe, was this a consensual encounter?

FINN. *(finally)* Yes. It was. I consented.

JAMES. *(exhaling)* Ok, that was . . . that was scary for a second.

FINN. Sorry, I didn't mean to scare you.

JAMES. No, no, I'm just glad you're ok!

FINN. And I'm sorry, about not using a condom.

JAMES. *(sinking)* Yeah, um, me too. I really wish you had. I feel like shit.

FINN. Me too, babe. I made a mistake. I don't really know how or why or what happened. I just wanted to be honest with you.

JAMES. Thanks. This really sucks.

FINN is silent. JAMES begins to cry. FINN can see this and tries to comfort them. It does not work. JAMES sets the phone face down, FINN begs them to return to the phone. JAMES takes the pancake plate and hurls it across the room. It shatters against the wall. FINN's pleas intensify. JAMES cleans up the pieces as the lights fade to black. In the dark FINN's pleas continue until they don't.

I was gonna call Finnegan twelve eggs because he dozen want me

(haha)

Imagine if I called him Eggs

(Eggs Benedict because he's a fucking traitor!!!!)

Finnegan as Eggs, a Short Poem Using Metaphors, Analogies, and a Common Theme of Poultry:

Scrambled: how my insides felt after fornication (yum)

Fried: because *damn* the sex was hot (close cousin of scrambled)

Over Easy: idk he seemed to get Over me Easy considering he literally married someone else six months later but we'll get to that

Poached: like what that fuck-ass man did, stealing my boyfriend

Soft-Scrambled: how I am softening about that other fuck-ass man because I am not about to reinforce the misogynistic homewrecker stereotype solely because I'm miffed. I may be miffed but anger should not come between me and my feminist agenda!!!! Let us not forget it was he, Finnegan, who chose to leave me!

Pickled: accepting I cannot blame that other fuck-ass man when Finnegan had full autonomy, but man oh man does it feel good to blame him

Deviled: how I felt hatching a plan to write a two-hundred-page literary diss track about him

Sunny-Side Up: realizing I didn't actually write this because I hated him, I needed to stop hating myself for something that wasn't my fault

Omelette: I'm-a-lette you imagine I tied this poem up nicely because we need to transition here

Back to my point, think about how it would seminally change this piece were I to call him "Eggs." For instance, compare and contrast the following passages:

It is a spring day, and I open my phone to scroll Instagram along with the millions of other millennials who stay connected to the outside world through the thin brick-size devices in our pockets. I toggle to my burner account and decide to stalk my ex, Finnegan. It is there I see a photo of Finnegan and a man I don't know. Finnegan is holding his hand. Both of them, including my ex Finnegan, are wearing wedding rings. In the background is the exact West Village location Finnegan claimed he wanted for our engagement. I cannot imagine Finnegan proposing to me now, just as I couldn't imagine Finnegan not proposing to me then. I am steamed, seeing this photo. It has been six months. I still bleed sometimes. And there it is, served to me on a platter, the very evidence Finnegan has run off with someone else. The very evidence Finnegan could easily toss me aside and move on. I feel my heart crack. I am a shell of a person. How embarrassing to think Finnegan wanted to be with me. How embarrassing to have been egged on by Finnegan's charm. How embarrassing to have a heart so heavy at the sight of Finnegan's engagement, but here we are. I close the burner account because I can't close the wound.

It is a spring day, and I open my phone to scroll Instagram along with the millions of other millennials who stay connected to the outside world through the thin brick-size devices in our pockets. I toggle to my burner account and decide to stalk my ex, Eggs. It is there I see a photo of Eggs and a man I don't know. Eggs is holding his hand. Both of them, including my ex Eggs, are wearing wedding rings. In the background is the exact West Village location Eggs claimed he wanted for our engagement. I cannot imagine Eggs proposing to me now, just as I couldn't imagine Eggs not proposing to me then. I am steamed, seeing this photo. It has been six months. I still bleed sometimes. And there it is, served to me on a platter, the very evidence Eggs has run off with someone else. The very evidence Eggs could easily toss me aside and move on. I feel my heart crack. I am a shell of a person. How embarrassing to think Eggs wanted to be with me. How embarrassing to have been egged on by Eggs's charm. How embarrassing to have a heart so heavy at the sight of Eggs's engagement, but here we are. I close the burner account because I can't close the wound.

Which one makes you want to go grab the nearest cage-free dozen and pelt his car in July? Which one makes you want to whisk him away and beat him in a mixing bowl? Which one makes you want to go virgin—I mean vegan—forever?

This has been a lesson in both poultry-themed literary devices, and how picking the wrong man can completely ruin your morning/life.

Over Hard: the realization that your former boyfriend is marrying someone else, which means he really doesn't love you anymore, and maybe he never did.

Eggs do not go well with pancakes, if you're wondering how the two proposal traumas fit together. One man I barely knew, who wanted me badly. I was too young. The other I thought I knew, but it turns out he didn't want me so badly. I was still young. Honestly, I still am.

It is a strange thing to have two proposals so cleanly permeate your orbit before twenty-five; one you got, one you didn't. Most of you probably forgot about the first proposal, the one with the blueberry pancakes and the fluffy cat and the "I don't even know your middle name" line, but my body certainly doesn't.

I'm not sure why breakfast food is the common theme here. I suppose it has to do with the first thing you want when you wake up in the morning.

#76–#84 8:30 p.m.
76th–84th Hookups After •••

I have been invited to an orgy probably because I'm super hot and sent really enticing bulge pics to the host, and I intend to capitalize on this opportunity by giving and getting as much dick as I can.

Sex parties in studio apartments are an operation, and luckily, I have Been Here and Done This. If you get there early enough (gays are always late, so this is to say if you get there even close to on time) you might be lucky enough to partake in the Preparation and Selection portion of the evening. I've met this host (#76) before, at another party (in my younger, un-raped days) so he invites me plenty early for Preparation and Selection. Auspicious beginning!

When I arrive, #76 buzzes me in, sporting hair down to his shoulders and a trimmed mustache. We kiss, I kick my shoes off, and settle on the couch next to him and three other boys I'll fuck later (#77, #78, and #79). For now we need to Prepare and Select. [Redacted cruising app that wouldn't be redacted if they'd answered my emails for a paid product placement in this book] is AirPlayed on the TV. We take turns pointing to various profiles and deliberating invitation offers.

I choose Asian 5'7" Vers Top, who becomes #80; the other boys pick a smattering of men (Otter 5'9" Loves Rimming; Black Dom; a faceless profile; and Geeky Top 7.5 Inches) who become #81–#84. There are nearly thirty invitees, but they do not get numbers because I did not have intercourse with them due to my nature as both highly selective and pure. They are simply sweaty background decorations, but it's important to know they're present and having lives of their own. Sex sonder, if you will.

#76, the host, has laid out a charcuterie board, and I've brought a bag of mints (never show up to someone's house empty-handed, and never let bad breath ruin the orgy!). #77 brought wet-wipe packs, and #78 brought cups and Sharpies because it is important to stay hydrated at these things (cum does not count).

One by one the men file in: Asian 5'7" Vers Top; the Otter; the Black Dom; the faceless profile who turns out to be a white bearded bear; the Geeky Top with his 7.5 Inches; and approximately thirty other irrelevant men whom I simply won't have time to fuck later but who are still hot and desirable nonetheless.

Soon enough I've kicked my clothes to a corner and #81 is kissing my neck, flanked by #76 on my backside. #77 is fondling #80 much to the enjoyment of a man watching from the couch. There is a bed at the center of the room, and #82 and a rando are slobbering all over each other like bulldogs. There are few words exchanged other than "mmm," "yum," and the ultra-common "fuuuuuck," so it sounds the way it feels: good. I am naked and being kissed and loved and worshipped and I feel safe because it would be really hard to rape me here given there are over thirty other men watching me and what's that saying? Safety in numbers? I have both: safety and numbers.

Because I'm a show-off (don't act surprised) I pull #76 onto the bed, flipping my legs up over his shoulders. #82 and the rando scoot over to make space (good orgy etiquette!). Before long a melisma of moans escapes my lips. I can feel multiple new eyes on me confirming that I am, indeed, the first penetration of the evening. #76 is sweet, he's going slow. I've picked him on purpose:

1. He's hot and I want to have sex with him
2. He's the host, and it's impolite not to have sex with the host at his own party
3. He's smaller than average, which is the perfect warm-up. I need durability if I'm to have half a dozen of these boys tonight, so I can't start out with the hung horses.*

A cluster of boys are watching #76 work me over, their knees slack from simultaneously pleasuring themselves. I notice #77's appendage is closest to me, so I flip over and take him in my mouth. I am now the first spitroast of the evening, which emits a chorus of "oh, fucks" and "that's hots," #78 gets brave and kneels on the bed next to #77. I switch my mouth from one cock to the other, rewarding his bravery. I hear another couple plop onto the bed next to me, and to make room

*This is a metaphor, to be clear. I do not fuck horses, that is bestiality, which is illegal, and this is not a production of *Equus*. Thank you.

I switch back to missionary. #76 has pulled out in the process. He smacks my ass, kisses me, and says he'll "be back."

#79 seizes the moment and says, "Can I?" lining up his dick up to the edge of the bed where my hips are easily accessible. I nod, #77 still in my mouth, and I see #80 line up behind #79. Lines at sex parties are my favorite thing, and I immediately harden. Lines mean that despite the dozens of other eligible suitors they could have in the meantime, they have decided to wait for you. It's the ultimate compliment, in my opinion. #80 must've seen me get hard because as #79 (notably bigger than #76) pushes in, he grabs my dick and begins to suck it.

ORGY NOTE: I've found "I'll be back" is a common and polite turn of phrase at orgies. It ends your time together without being rude (so many men, so little time!), and affirms that you enjoyed the experience. Occasionally they do, indeed, come back, but even if they don't, you're ideally occupied by someone else. After all, no one goes to an orgy to have sex with one singular person the entire time!

I am now where I was born to be: taking one dick in either end while mine gets sucked. It does not get better than this. I feel fantastic.

#79 trades places with #80 until he gets distracted by someone else and parts ways. #80 is going at it hard, but he's exactly the right size so it doesn't hurt.

"I like your nails," he says, and I remember mine are painted pink.

"Thank you." I smile and let #77 flop out of my mouth. He pats my cheek affectionately and hoists himself off the bed.

"Your femininity is so hot." It's #80 again, who has taken a break from thrusting to offer a compliment that careens right into all my insecurities.

"Thank you." I nearly blush as I sit up. He grabs at my bun, tied precariously with two hair ties. His grip feels great.

"Woof." He grins. I look into his eyes, satin black, and kiss him. He kisses me back with a light hair pull. I growl, and he pushes me back on the bed. My head accidentally knocks against #81's knee, which was apparently in mid-dismount from the mattress.

"Oh, sorry babe!" #81 says, cupping my head in his hands. "Are you ok?" His legs are a V on either side of my ears. His leg hair is soft. I am most certainly ok. "Oh, wow," he says, still holding my head. "You're so cute."

I giggle, looking up at his buzzed head and young eyes. "Thanks, so are you." I reach up and knot my fingers into his chest hair, pulling him over me. "Kiss me," I say. He does, tongue first. His mouth tastes like one of the random guys I won't fuck that evening. It's hot because he's with me now, not them.

"Can I coach you?" he breathes into my mouth.

"Oh, absolutely."

The coaching is hot, intense, and the whole time #81 is cradling my head in his hands. There is a misnomer about doms or verbally intensive guys being rough or aggressive, and while they certainly can be (with consent!), #81's otter fingers were soft against my temples the entire time. It was grounding. Soothing, even.

I notice #82, the Black Dom, watching me from the corner of the room. I wink at him. He grabs his balls and winks back. #81 is still coaching me, he'll have to wait.

#81 finishes our session by trading places with #79, at which point he is so hard and so close that he comes almost instantly. Sweat falls from his brow onto my belly, and he heaves through his orgasm. Being the bottom someone decides to deposit into at an orgy is also an honor—for most men, once they cum, they're done. So if they decide to end with you, it's a compliment. I sit up again, smile, and make space for someone else to get railed on my corner of the bed.

ORGY NOTE: Coaching is exactly what you think it is—it's when a man (like #81) decides to tell the other top (in this case, #79) how to fuck you whilst also telling the bottom (in this case, yours truly) how to take it. It often includes phrases like "Yeah, enjoy that boypussy" and "Take his big cock, tell me how much you like it." It's a derivative of the verbal kink that I'm pretty sure originates in the jock / athlete / fucking-your-coach-in-the-locker-room-to-stay-on-the-team type of porn, but is easily translatable to many mediums such as masturbation groups, Zoom sex rooms, and in this case, orgies with #81 and #79.

"That was hot," I tell #81, who is still catching his handsome otter breath.

"Yeah, wow." He grabs my right butt cheek. "It definitely was. I'm gonna . . ." He motions to the counter where he will retrieve a wet wipe before dressing and exiting. He will have to navigate the tangle of bodies pleasuring each other in the middle of the room to get there, but that's part of the fun.

I send him off. "See you later!"

#79 is downing a glass of water on the other side of the room. He sees that I'm free, and motions to the cups and then at me with a raised brow.

I nod vigorously. Yes, I would love some water right now. He and #81 counter each other as they traverse the twister pile, and I make eye contact with #82 who is also making his way over.

"Here you go." #79 hands me the cup of water. I chug it.

"Thank you so much," I exhale. "I needed that!"

"Yeah, you were working hard." He pauses. "Could I possibly get your number before I go? I'd like to see you again."

"Yeah, totally!" I nod and set my cup down on the shelf to my right before looping my bun into place.

"Awesome, I'll go grab my phone. Be right back."

He disappears into the boypit right as #82 lands next to me. He's so tall that I have to look up at him.

"Well, hello there." My head is tilted forty-five degrees north.

"Hi," he greets me with a hand around my throat. I harden. "You like that?"

"Yes, sir," I say, and he pushes me back onto the bed where I belong.

His third leg is truly a third leg (enormous), but #79 and #76 have opened me up, so I'm confident I can take it. Someone holds a bottle of poppers to my nose and I take a whiff, grateful they noticed the challenge I was about to take on. God, I love power.

#82 isn't a rougher dom than #81, he's just bigger (which feels rougher), but too many people are watching for me to quit. Plus, I hadn't seen #82 inside anyone else all night, and my desire for exceptionalism widens my hole. (At least that's what I tell myself.) #82 pins my shoulders down and pounds me into the mattress.

At some point I see #79, phone in hand, in my peripheral vision. My back stiffens, afraid someone is filming me, but then I remember #79 had asked for my number, but #82 had grabbed me before we could follow through. #79 looked caught.

"Hey," I say to #82, my voice vibrating with his thrusting. "He asked for my number, can I—"

#82 looks at #79 and waves him over with a nod, never breaking his rhythm. I'm impressed. I hold on to #82's bulging biceps with my left arm and take #79's phone with my right. #82 is going so hard I can't see the screen straight. One by one I press my phone number into his contacts, hoping my thumb hasn't slipped amidst the intense fucking.*

"Thanks, err, have a good night!" #79 looks like he wants to kiss me, but with a glance from #82 he backs away.

"How's it feel?" #82 asks me, completely focused on my face.

"Amazing,"

"I'm getting close," he says, and I can feel him go even harder.

I grip his triceps, a fan favorite. "Yeah?"

He moans, and I take my second load of the night.

This time when I sit up my core hurts and my head goes light, usually a sign of a deep dicking. He helps me up and rubs my shoulders.

"Your hole is amazing."

"Thank you." I kiss him, and realize it's our first kiss. I'd let this man ejaculate inside me before we so much as locked lips. Group sex is funny that way.

"I'm gonna go clean off," I say with a final arm squeeze. "You felt really good too."

I am cleaning myself with a wad of wet wipes when I lock eyes with #83, the faceless-profile-turned-bearded-bear. He is being rimmed by a white boy I'd seen but not linked with yet. The bear beckons me over, and I smile. On my way I pass #84, the Geeky Top whose 7.5 inches are inside a different white guy who must've just arrived, given that his underwear is only halfway down his calves. Our eyes meet. I kiss him, he keeps fucking the newbie.

"Hi." I bite his ear playfully.

"Hellooooo," he says, sliding his thumb inside my mouth. I close my lips around it and suck.

"Oh fuuuuck," he breathes. The newbie squeals below him, no doubt thinking he is responsible for his top's sudden outburst. I place a hand on the newbie's back, gently coaxing him to arch further. He does, with an "Oh, man." #84's eyes roll back.

"Come find me next," I whispered in #84's ear, and move toward #83. The bear had been abandoned by his rimmer and was waiting eagerly.

"Do you want to fuck me?" he says, and it dawns on me that I haven't topped tonight.

* To this day I'm worried I messed up, seeing as how #79 still hasn't texted me.

"Absolutely, what position do you want to be in?"

He replies by climbing onto the bed and arching his ass toward me. He is the right height for me to insert without bending my knees.

"Oh, you're so thick," he says, among a slew of other affirmatives I won't write for fear of making you all deeply attracted to me.

I start slow, and when he signals for more, I go for it. Sometimes at orgies if I've touched myself or been touched enough I can plateau and remain hard for extended periods of time without cumming or softening. It's like an environmentally induced Viagra, and lucky for #83 I am in that phase. I grab his hips and keep going. He is loving it.

I feel warmth behind me, and a pair of hands lands on either side of us, accompanied by a nibble at my ear.

"Hey, sexy." It's the Geeky Top, #84. "Can I?" He pushes his uncircumcised tip against me.

"Please do." And before I'd finished the sentence every last inch had disappeared inside me.

I crane my neck to face #84. "Go for it," I say and with a smile he dials it up to jackhammer and I boomerang in and out of #83. I am moaning, #83 is moaning, everyone is moaning. #84 puts his hands past me onto #83's hips to push his 7.5 inches even deeper, which I did not think possible until I felt it. He slaps against me over and over and over and I feel like a goddess, sandwiched in between two beautiful men who both clearly want me very badly.

And suddenly #84 stops. I sniff, wondering if I've had an accident. I don't smell anything, but his response is alarming.

"Um . . ." #84's hands are on my back, and he's looking down, examining.

ORGY NOTE: Now, if you've never experienced a three-way like this before, when you're in the middle of two boys in this position, it usually goes one of two ways:

1) You, the one in the middle, do all the work. You are doing the fucking and fucking yourself simultaneously. You control speed, tempo, angle, thrusting, everything, which can be helpful, especially if the position is new. Since you're literally topping and bottoming at the same time, you want to make sure you listen to your own bodily cues as well as stay attuned to your bottom's. Mine is relaxing his lumbar so I know he is good. Freedom of movement is often indicative of comfort.

2) The top inside you does all the work, and the momentum of his thrust (and its reverb) pushes you in and out of your bottom. He has to use enough force to essentially double fuck: you into your bottom and back into you. It's intense, but oh so hot if you're able to accomplish it. Tonight? I am gonna try.

"What?" I soften with fear inside #83.

"I think you're—"

"Oh, shit, am I not clean anymore?" I reach a hand between my legs for the small traces of fecal matter I expect to find but my fingers reach a different wetness just as he says,

"I think you're bleeding."

"Oh fuck, Jesus, sorry!" I pull out of #83 as gingerly as I can, my heart racing.

"No, it's ok!" #84 was concerned. "Are you hurt?"

"No, no, it doesn't hurt." I clench my cheeks and turn toward the bathroom on the other side of the apartment. "I'm just sorry I bled on you!"

"It happens, I'm sorry if I went too hard or—"

"It's not you at all, don't even worry." I make the mistake of glancing down at his penis, which is sheathed in a thin layer of scarlet liquid. I am horrified.

By some miracle the bathroom is free. I lock the door behind me and clamber onto the toilet. I feel it slither out of me, the blood, gooped up by lube and semen. I don't look into the bowl, I bunch up toilet paper and press it against my hole. The paper stings.

Suddenly it is a midnight in October, I am in my shower, and I'm bleeding. My voice is hoarse from saying, "No, please stop," to a man who wasn't Finn, so when the blood comes my cries are silent. I sink down into the tub and watch the blood spool out of me like a ribbon dancer, slinking across the porcelain center and slipping down the drain. I want Finnegan. I want anything but this.

Then I'm back in #76's apartment, sweating, holding a wad of bright red toilet paper. The nails #79 liked so much glitter pink at the perimeter.

I cannot be this girl. I cannot be the girl who bled on everyone at the sex party. I cannot be the girl who bled on everyone at the sex party and cries in the bathroom after being triggered because of something that happened far too long ago. I cannot move, despite the sweat under my thighs threatening to spill me from atop the toilet. I stare at the paper wad, red seeping to its corners, crumpled like hibiscus petals in my fist. I was doing so well.

I can't go back and face #84. I'm so embarrassed. One moment I was in ecstasy and the next I'm bleeding all over his dick like a fucking loser. I don't want to see him or anyone else. I want to jump out the window and run. I want to stop crying. I want to stop every stupid fluid in my body from spilling out of me against my will. I stay, squeezing my hole over the toilet, until I hear a rap at the door.

"Just a minute!" I say, and it sounds like a lie.

It's a lie because it has been more than a minute. It has been more minutes than I care to count—countless, even—and no matter how hard I try I'm still in pain.

Around the same time Peter Hanson boarded United Airlines Flight 175 from Boston to LA I was getting dropped off at school. He would've passed through the Logan terminal and slung his luggage onto the security conveyor belt around the same time I would've slung my backpack onto my desk to remove a few pencils for the morning assignment. He would've picked it back up on the other end of the X-ray machine and meandered toward the terminal just as I would've skipped my way down the courtyard to my second class of the day. He would've rounded the corner to his gate just as I rounded the corner to the music classroom. As he shuffled onto the aircraft with fifty-five other passengers, seven flight attendants, and two pilots, I would've scurried into music class with twenty-eight other kindergarteners accompanied by one teacher and one teacher's aide. We called these classes "Specials"—art, music, physical education, and other forms of enrichment whose funding was consistently threatened by an ever-greedy and knuckleheaded flock of balding bureaucrats. Peter probably would've considered his airport excursion "special" as well. He was on his way to Disneyland.

While I was thumping out the bass section of "Hot Cross Buns" on an oversize Orff instrument with an accompanying yarn-headed mallet, Peter would witness two men stab a flight attendant, deploy an irritant spray, and overtake the cockpit of the plane. How they managed to enter is unknown, considering FAA rules require doors to remain closed and locked during flight, similar to how I don't remember the order of events that put me alone in the back closet with Mr. Anderson later that morning.

We can assume the hijackers threatened the flight crew with their weapons, demanding them to open the door, just as it makes the most sense that Mr. Anderson told my teacher I had "musical promise" and he wanted a few extra moments to assess, deploying his weapon of choice: a charming grin.

During the ordeal Peter Hanson made two phone calls, both to his father. In the first one, he said:

> *I think they've taken over the cockpit—an attendant has been stabbed—and someone else up front may have been killed. The plane*

is making strange moves. Call United Airlines—tell them it's Flight 175, Boston to LA.

Hanson's plane would've hooked back toward New York City as I would've handed the first round of Orffs to Mr. Anderson. Clean-Up Crew was a coveted position because it meant you were trusted to handle the instruments, which is to say you were trusted with the safety of music itself. I had already been playing piano for two years. I loved music, I loved nothing more than being trusted with packing up the Orffs, I felt immense pride as I plucked mallets from the ground and returned them to the comfort of their cases in the massive closet.

At this time, I would've been so small that my feet wouldn't touch the ground in an aircraft seat, so I doubt I was really much assistance to Mr. Anderson when putting away the large, percussive blocks, but he let me do it anyway. It gave me purpose, it made me feel important, and most of all it made me feel like a grown-up.

The youngest 9/11 victim happened to be seated next to Peter: Christine Hanson, his daughter. She had tottered through security with her father and mother, Sue Kim, and boarded Flight 175. I imagine she was excited; it was her first time on an airplane. Christine was two and a half years old.

Back in the music classroom, at some point Mr. Anderson's pants fall like the towers; you know the rest.

Christine had recently been gifted her favorite stuffed animal, Peter Rabbit, by her grandmother, Eunice. I can only assume this stuffed animal was not on board Flight 175 because Eunice and her husband, Lee, donated it to the 9/11 museum in 2014. I visited when I found out. I don't know why. 2014 was the same year I found the memorial lights, my first year of college, my first year as a New Yorker. I had kissed only two boys, hadn't come into myself as trans, hadn't lived away from home, hadn't even had sex yet. I don't know why I went; I think I just wanted to pay my respects.

Peter Rabbit was in a glass case in the left rear wing of the museum. He's still there, you can find him. I visited again while writing this and noticed something new: two Pooh Bear stickers on Peter Rabbit's torso are still attached. They furl at the edges, revealing bits of fuzz clinging to the backing. "She put stickers on everything she liked," I remember Eunice saying in an interview.

I had an intense emotional reaction accompanying this realization; these Pooh Bear stickers are the same age as my sexual trauma. They still cling to the rabbit fur twenty years later, memorialized in a glass case so no one can touch.

In the same interview Eunice said she imagined all of Christine's milestones: her first day of kindergarten, her high school graduation, her first job out of college. "You go through all these wonders," she said. "And then I get angry with those people that did this awful murder."

I am angry too. I am angry that at the time of this book's publication, Christine would've been twenty-six but she isn't because she was murdered. I'm angry that 9/11 became an excuse for horrific Islamophobia, racism, and an upsurge of American fascism branded as "patriotism." I am angry that I know people who had to move jobs—even countries—because they were scrutinized and ridiculed after 9/11 for their race or religion. I am angry that people do not understand that the enemy of our enemy sometimes is our friend, if only in idea and politic, not execution, and I am angry that the same cops who brutalize Black people in our streets were hailed as heroes in the weeks following 9/11. I am angry that 81 percent of women in this country report being sexually assaulted or harassed in their lifetime, and that 33 percent of them report it happening between the ages of eleven and seventeen, which means that if Christine were alive it is more possible than not she would resonate with the general theme of this book. I am angry I even have to write that sentence, because I know how atrocious it sounds, and I am angry that someone will miss the point entirely and think I'm capitalizing off someone's murder for my own gain rather than pointing out we seem to care a whole hell of a lot about people in theory, but fail to protect them when they're actually alive. How many Christines have grown up in a society that harasses and assaults them, only to victim-blame and disbelieve them after, and why aren't more people angry alongside me?

I look at Peter Rabbit, and I remember Peter Hanson's final phone call:

It's getting bad, Dad—a stewardess was stabbed—they seem to have knives and Mace—they said they have a bomb—it's getting very bad on the plane—passengers are throwing up and getting sick—the plane is making jerky movements—I don't think the pilot is flying the plane—I think we are going down—I think they intend to go to Chicago or someplace and fly into a building—don't worry, Dad—if it happens, it'll be very fast . . .

Mr. Anderson is in the back closet, looking at me, flanked by the instruments I've gathered. He peers his head around the doorframe. The classroom is empty, the Orffs have long ceased sound making. He looks at me, asks if I want to see something, and I nod. It will be more instruments, a cooler Orff, maybe even a marimba. Instead he unfastens the top button.

". . . Don't worry . . . it'll be very fast . . ."

It was. It was fast. He was right. What everyone forgets is that the speed of the action does not dictate the impact of the trauma. It takes a split second for a plane to fly into a building, killing thousands of people, among them a two-year-old girl. It takes only a split second for your music teacher to molest you amidst the instruments from that day's lesson.

But the aftermath? It isn't fast. Not for me, not for Eunice, not for every living Christine trying to navigate this world without becoming a statistic.

It clings to us, like Pooh Bear stickers.

Finn, Before

Finnegan was the first person to call it a boob.

We were tucked into my bed sometime after I'd met his friends and before he left for the other side of the world, and I asked him:

"What's your favorite position?"

"The one where I'm inside you."

"No!" I elbowed him. "I mean like to cuddle in."

The angles of him layered on top of me like transparency sheets on a projector. His nose pressed the flesh behind my earlobe. I colored the wall with the anticipation in my breath. Under the pillow I could see the hair stake its claim around the bones of his wrist. I was afraid I was crushing his forearm, but more afraid of separating his nose from my ear to ask.

His free fingers found the space in between mine, curling into my palm. In return I closed mine on top of his. We were holding hands. He had initiated it. No finger guns, just fingers. The wall reminded me to keep breathing.

"I guess this is what I usually go for," he said. I could tell his eyes were closed.

"This position?"

"Well, more like this, actually," He switched our arms so his snaked underneath mine. His fingertips pulled a tributary across my chest, settling into the crook of my armpit, my nipple webbed in the lattice of his palm.

"I like going for the boob." His scruff tickled my neck. I giggled. "It gives me something to hold."

My chest, at the time, was flat, nothing material to hold, yet something stirred in the fibers beneath his hand. The wall and I attributed it to love or lust or falling for him; now I would attribute to affirmation. It was as if his hand on my body and that word in my ear tied two loose strings together that I'd been tripping over. The lines in his palm tugged at the breast tissue that would be built years later off little blue pills and memories of my mother's heels, T-shirts on my head, the letter *s* added to my former pronoun.

Girlhood was something more than the need to be fucked or the itch to grow my hair out or $80 at the nail salon "because I like how it looks," it was something that could be held. I let him hold it. I can't say for how long. I can say it became my favorite position, too.

It was his doctor's idea to write the daily schedule on a whiteboard for him, and our idea to write down all the names of his family members. It was my idea to add pictures. Now, usually in the mornings, we quiz him: Who's that? *(My father.)* And what about him? *(My uncle.)* And this person? *(My cousin.)*

Today we are running him through the painstaking ritual of ensuring us he hasn't declined to the point of forgetting his extended family when he trips up on one of my cousins. He is saying she is my aunt. In fairness, they do look similar, but if the dementia residue has hardened to plaque in the corners of your brain that denote time frame you might confuse my cousin for my aunt because you think it's 1998. My grandmother is visibly upset and puts the whiteboard aside. He can sense something is wrong, and he goes to pick up the board.

"No, leave it." She kisses his cheek. "We don't need to do that right now."

"Well, what do we need to do?" The last vowel has a shadow that originates in the hills of Kentucky.

At least he won't lose his accent, I think, and remember it is entirely possible he will die nonverbal, as so many others with this disease. I return to cutting his strawberries and toss them into the dollop of yogurt swirled with his favorite granola.

"This is ready," I say, handing the bowl to my grandmother across the high-top ledge.

"Oh, wonderful, look at this!" She shows him the bowl.

"Good deal!" He grabs a spoon, proving instinct has not left him completely, perhaps only temporarily misplaced.

"You." He cranes his neck to see me abandon the kitchen to land in his line of vision. "You are a very helpful young man!"

Man.

"Thank you." I laugh. "Enjoy your breakfast."

"Do you know who that is?" My grandmother asks him. He is quiet.

"Well, of course!"

"Who is it?"

"That's James, our grandson."

"Yes, yes it is! Good deal." I slide her a bowl of her own yogurt. We share a look.

James, my grandson.

I am relieved to be misgendered for perhaps the first time in my life because at least I am still known. He gets a pass because he is losing memories every day and I would rather him hold on to a half-truth than lose all concept of me completely. He will be the last person ever allowed to call me his grandson or use masculine honorifics to describe me. And when he dies that part of my gender will die with him, or he'll take the remnants of it, if they're not too much to carry, to wherever he is going next.

#92 11:29 a.m.
92nd Hookup After

92: [sends four pictures all of which scream, in order, "the gods have favorites and I'm one of them" and "you couldn't carve more muscle on these six-feet-three-inches if you tried," followed up with "my smile is also particularly dashing underneath this mustache" and "I have a Doberman and she is the Bestest Girl"]

J: oh woooofffff

J: [insert series of photos that say "with respect to your dog I am temporarily challenging her for who can be the Bestest Girl"]

92: yes please baby

J: oof call me that and you're gonna get exactly what you want

92: oh is that so?

92: . . . baby?

J: oohhhh yeah

J: what're you into?

92: [long explicit list of sexual tastes, kinks, and fetishes ranging from mild vanilla to intensive BDSM]

J: [eagerly chooses a collection of experiences tailored toward the more vanilla side because I am feeling emotionally fragile and femme today and not quite ready to be in a sub space despite being conceptually willing to do anything for the marble-sculpture of a man messaging me his nudes]

92: I'd love to do all that with you baby boy

92: treat you right

J: [deciding to be brave!!!] actually not a boy :)

92: oh sorry

92: baby girl

92: or baby they

J: hahah baby they I've never heard that before

J: kinda cute tbh

J: baby girl also works if you're down?

92: yeah I'm bi I don't discriminate

J: well I think you're really hot and I def wanna be your baby girl / baby they if you're free

92: yeah, you travel?

J: exclusively

92: [insert address]

J: awesome be there in 20

The photos are right, the gods do have favorites, and he is definitely one of them. I was wrong about the height though; he is a clean six feet five, and I'm really trying not to have a height thing but when you're trying to be the Bestest Girl (Doberman be damned) it is useful when the man on about to be on top of you is twice your size in most directions.

"Hi, baby they." His mustache tickles me on the downswing of his kiss. I laugh into his lips.

"Hi, daddy," I volley. His hand finds the back of my neck.

"Mm, that's right."

The sex is surprisingly good. Despite the warm lead-up I am nervous; muscle hunks have a reputation for spending more time pumping creatine into their system than learning how to be considerate partners, and I had tempered my expectations of #92 with this fact. It is perhaps the reason I find myself more consistently attracted to the Dad Bod than the Muscle Gay—I've never met one of the latter who cared more about the human in front of them than their own physique.

#92 has the makings of an exception. We fuck like animals—he literally growls at me during foreplay, which I find delicious and dangerously sexy. He knows how to warm me up, he knows how to cater his body to the position that makes me most comfortable, we even do it standing because everything lines up between my giraffe legs and his meat-packed six-foot-five stilts. The mirror in his apartment is exquisitely placed so I can watch him watch me be the Bestest Girl. The Doberman licks my foot at one point and we both have to stop to laugh. Sex is funny. It's silly. We are aimless animals mashing our genitals together to feel something: connection, pleasure, worthiness.

And with #92 I am connected, I feel pleasure, I feel worth his time. He is certainly worth mine, which he makes apparent by offering to bottom for me knowing full well flipping is my favorite. He says he hasn't bottomed in a while but "just can't resist that cock," which I find to be a wholly understandable sentiment.

He has a meeting on the hour, so I don't stay long after climax. I do not cry; in fact I am fine with this. I had managed to steer clear of sub space whilst having a thoroughly satisfying and exciting afternoon of intercourse. I kiss his mustache again, and I hop out the door.

4:36 p.m.:

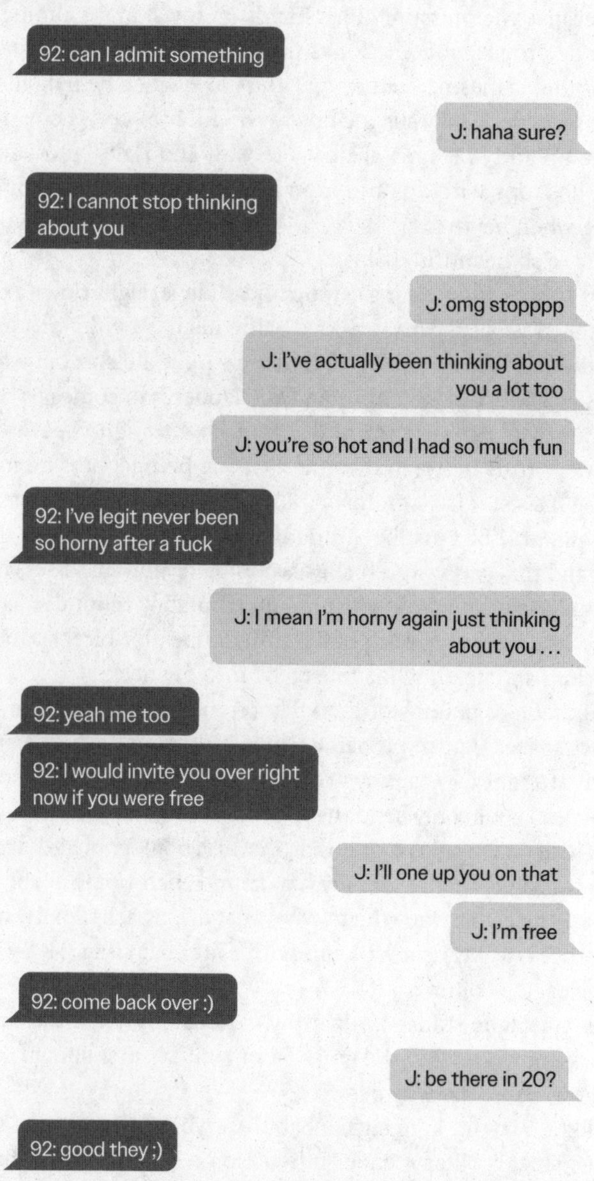
92: can I admit something
J: haha sure?
92: I cannot stop thinking about you
J: omg stopppp
J: I've actually been thinking about you a lot too
J: you're so hot and I had so much fun
92: I've legit never been so horny after a fuck
J: I mean I'm horny again just thinking about you . . .
92: yeah me too
92: I would invite you over right now if you were free
J: I'll one up you on that
J: I'm free
92: come back over :)
J: be there in 20?
92: good they ;)

The second time is even better. The mustache scratches an itch I need against my lip, my hole, maybe my heart. I love the way he paws at me because the pressure of his hands on my skin is calming, I love the way he growls while he looks me in the eyes like he equal parts owns me and is mesmerized by me, and I love when he puts his knees over my shoulders and tells me how well I fill him up. At one point he picks me up and holds me against the wall and right before he reenters me he stops with an abruption that makes me think something is wrong when he says:

"You're so beautiful, baby girl."

And I think I'll melt into syrup and slide straight down the wall, a sappy, sticky, sugary mess. I love being his baby girl—or I just love that he didn't see me as a boy. Both. It feels right, I'll sort out why later.

We finish. I cum, he cums, and the Doberman comes to ball herself at our feet. I try not to think about how I might weave into his life; grocery runs between meetings for the bell peppers he forgot or following his sister back on Instagram or dancing to live jazz music on a Friday night. I had just begun reminding myself that all of this was fantasy and this was only a fuck—two unbelievably good sets of fucks in a singular day, at that—when he interrupts my reminder by rolling on top of me, scooping both of his cantaloupes-for-biceps around my midsection, and nestling his mustache into my neck.

Hundreds of pounds of hunk lay on me, his paws at the back of my heart-space. He can probably feel it kick from both sides. I make a valiant attempt to wrap my arms around him, but restricted by the cantaloupes I could only bend them at the elbow and the wrist, making strange scalene triangles that hover over his shoulder blades. I look like a T. rex. I change tactics and my hands find their home at the base of his spine. The ceiling fan whirrs. My sweat drips back into my hairline. He breathes out. My nose balloons with a familiar sting. My eyes ready themselves. It's coming.

His mustache ruffles against my earlobe, and he kisses it with a lightness known only to the grass from winter's first snowflake.

"Wow, baby," he whispers.

And he is right, I am such a baby. A crybaby who cannot seem to have one single solitary tender interaction without welling up. In my defense, there is something sacred about a top lying on your chest, especially after he's let you inside of him, and I have an entire personal weighted blanket of a top on top of me. I wish he would slide one of his paws up to cup my breast (with him they are breasts!). A surprising portion of me is willing to forfeit any sense of gender if it means I can be his; his good boy, his good girl, his good they, whatever kinky energy ends with bell peppers and followbacks and jazz clubs and him, lying on me, like this, pressing down so the hurt can't bubble up, regulating my system after wall-fucking and ear kisses and by the time I am done wanting this the wetness has started on my face.

It is challenging to cry in secret with a man this heavy on top of you because you have little margin of error for things like shuddering and I am a big shudderer when I cry. It starts about three-quarters of the way through once my parasympathetic nervous system pumps the Calm Down hormones through my synaptic pathways, at which point I'm terrified he'll catch this "hot babe with a tight body and a tight ass" (his words, earlier, second round against the wall) being loose and undesirable and scrunch-faced and snotty, but that's what I get for pushing it too far and wanting too much of a good thing.

His Doberman unfurls her tail and looks up at me with black eyes as if to say, "You tried, but I'll always be his Bestest Girl." She trots to his side of the bed, prying his attention from me with whimpers and whines, like she is mimicking every sound I made against the wall not fifteen minutes ago. He shushes her with one hand, the perfect opportunity to play my shudders off as laughs.

At two minutes till his next meeting, I scramble back into my clothes with record alacrity. I leave thinking I was wrong; she is the Bestest Girl, distracting him just enough for me to hide my tears. A dog can be a girl's girl, I suppose, even if I'm only partially a girl (but in the cute and sexy way #92 seems to like). I take the win. I need it.

We have hospice nurses now. They come to the house and check his vitals, and it surprises me how this does not make the situation any better. We thought the extra pairs of hands—or the presence of someone with medical expertise—might alleviate some of the burden, but we spend more time teaching them how to care for him than they do caring for him. We are beginning to wonder why we have called them in.

It was the pain. His, not ours. My grandfather has an infamously high pain tolerance; the fall that twisted his femur like a spiral cheese stick and confined him to this wheelchair resulted in two broken vertebrae, unbeknownst to us. It was not until a month into physical therapy that he mentioned back pain, and upon further examination by an X-ray machine, L1 and L2 were indeed broken. This was back in the earlier stages of Alzheimer's (Stage 2, Very Mild Cognitive Decline), when it was a fair question to ask how long he'd been in pain.

"Well, at least a month!" His spine had been broken the entire time and he had never once complained.

All of this to say, when he told us last week that his stomach hurt, we took it seriously. Action was taken. His doctors recommended hospice. We are waiting for them to be of use.

"His vitals are normal, but he does seem to be in a lot of pain," says a stethoscope-adorned woman so frazzled I shudder to think what her kitchen looks like.

"Do you have any idea what the problem could be?" my grandmother asks. We are both ready for the truth: His digestive system is shutting down, his body is waning, he is preparing to die.

"I'm afraid not. Could he have eaten anything that might have disagreed with his stomach?"

"No, ma'am, he hasn't eaten in days."

She fluffs her red hair as if the answer might be within the nest of coils. "Maybe the pain is because he needs to eat. Have you fed him?"

"Have we *fed him?*" My grandmother's incredulity slips past the flimsy barrier built on two hours of sleep.

"With all due respect"—my customer service voice is coming out—"we have tried to feed him multiple times today, yesterday, and the day before and he isn't interested. He sleeps sixteen hours a day at minimum now, and I'm sure the lethargy and the lack of appetite are connected, but this is out of character for him. I cook him meals every night and historically he eats everything I give him—he's always had a healthy appetite—so I'm wondering if there's anything else you can check or anything else you can d—"

"I totally get your concern, Mr. Rose"—*I hate her and her entire family*—"but sometimes this is what happens."

"So, does that mean this is the end? Or the end is near?" My grandmother looks at her.

"It's hard to say." The nurse takes us in. "I'll tell you what, I have a pack of morphine in the car with me."

"Morphine?"

"Yes. We often give it to patients experiencing extreme pain toward the end of their lives, especially when they are unwilling or unable to eat."

We are silent. The nurse excuses herself. My grandfather is lumped up in his sheets, eyes closed. The humidifier gurgles near the hallway. One of the red birds flits toward the window, but lands just out of view.

Finn, Before

The first time I met Finnegan I was a wreck. It was summer in New York, which meant I was dripping through my button-down, which was printed with tiny (wet) whales of assorted shades of blue. I forgot my pomade when I switched bags after the gym, and I was willing my coif not to droop in the cocktail of sweat and swelter. The A train stalled at Columbus Circle, and I was already six minutes late to the cookie shop on the corner of Forty-Fifth and Ninth where I was supposed to meet him. I had never been this late, this moist, or this nervous.

I reminded myself that nerves were irrational. We had talked every night for the past eleven days, notably the eleven days leading up to his New York arrival. I knew about his strained relationship with his father, and I'd seen the baby pictures where his mother was dipping his two-year-old toes into the ocean. I'd heard all the drama with his college roommates, and his last job. He told me he'd been single for the past year and he wasn't looking for something serious, but he couldn't stop thinking about me. I knew his astrological chart. I knew what his dick looked like. I knew exactly where to prop my laptop so it looked like he was lying next to me in bed. Still, we'd never actually met.

I dodged a taxi as I scurried across Forty-Sixth Street. I was less than a block away. I could have hurled. The cookie shop was two doors into the avenue, which was capped by a 5 Napkin Burger and a bevy of bicycles. I stood on the east side of Ninth Avenue, which meant I was one WALK signal and three traffic lanes away from seeing, kissing, touching, smelling, *meeting* an entire real-life Finnegan.

I wanted to know what he smells like, what his stubble would feel like brushing under my thumb. I wanted to know whether he shifts his weight to one side when he stands and how limp his wrists are in public. I wanted to know how well he tips servers at restaurants and how fast he walks and how big his hand would be measured against mine. I knew he'd be there, on the corner of Forty-Fifth and Ninth outside the cookie shop, but I couldn't move. I pulled out my phone and called him.

He picked up on the second ring. "What's up, babe?"

"I'm across the street," I managed, wiping my brow.

"Okay, so . . . cross the street, silly!" I could hear the same cars whizzing past through his phone.

I studied the ground, uneven asphalt stained with blackened gum. "I'm scared," I admitted.

"Of what?"

"What if you're ugly?"

"Oh, shut up and cross the street so I can meet you."

"You promise you're not ugly?"

"GoodBYE!"

I laughed, which brought with it a full breath. The light changed, and I crossed the street while the sun dripped onto the tips of the skyscrapers behind me. I passed the 5 Napkin Burger, the first door, and there he was, smiling and holding a bag of cookies. There must have been dozens of people passing us by, but I don't remember a single one. All of me was melting, inside and out, like a warm chocolate chip cookie in the palm of a seven-year-old. I remember his khaki shorts, hems tickling the tops of his knees. I remember his lips; rose pink, parted like an orange slice. I remember his hair; blond, loose locks dangling above his eyes. I remember his eyes; oceans at high tide, rich with diamonds, the color of a glacier as it rolls over in the Arctic sea. I remember my heart beating so fast I was afraid it would knock him clean across the avenue when he hugged me. He fit his arms around my rib cage, bag of cookies at my back.

"Hi, baby." His whisper drowned out New York City.

"I'm so happy," I said. He pulled away and studied my face. I felt every bead of sweat corrode what remained of my confidence. He kissed my cheek, stubble to stubble, inches from my lips.

"Me too."

I led him downtown for our first real-life, in-person date, and all the while he laughed at my ridiculous jokes, cookie bag swinging above the concrete. I am sure tourists and delivery workers on bicycles and theater patrons dodged us, the oblivious couple, cursing our lack of awareness, but I didn't notice. We found ourselves somewhere in the West Village, and we must've eaten at some point, but I don't remember the specifics. I remember the fireworks in my chest and I remember tumbling back onto the street and realizing the cookies had melted in the summer heat.

I remember the laughter, reverberating off the cobblestones, growing like weeds through the cracks.

On our way to the train I couldn't help but imagine how many times this street had carried new lovers through their first conversation, how many first kisses this slab of sidewalk had claimed, or this one, or this one, or this one. I wondered how many times that restaurant booth had heard the words *I'd really like to see you again*, or that barstool witnessed someone saying *Can I buy you a drink?* I wondered if the lights strung from one side of the street to another, hanging above our heads like fireflies, ever tired of couples holding hands and passing under them, pausing for a photo. I wished the bricks in the brownstones could tell me whether love actually made your feet lighter or it just felt that way. I wanted to ask the street signs if they knew how it would end or if they enjoyed the beginnings too much to care. Instead, I asked Finn to come back to my place. He said yes.

It was almost dark. Above us, the Sun was retiring for the evening, pulling the last of her colors into the Hudson River. The Moon was slipping out of her slumber, cresting in between the avenues, readying the tide to change. The Sun stopped, looked over her gleaming, buttery shoulder, and said to the Moon, "Watch this."

Below, two lovers kissed for the first time on the corner of Cornelia and Bleecker.

The Moon watched, and winked at the Sun, who had gathered the last of her oranges and pinks and slipped into the sea. The Moon turned away from the lovers, thinking to herself, "It'll never happen like that again." She unhooked gravity from her tool belt and went back to pulling the tide in from the shore. As she did, she dropped a flurry of gravity from the hole in her pocket and onto the lovers, binding one's heart to the other. It would chill them like cold wind and warm them like desire. They would later call it love.

I just couldn't take my eyes off him.

Morphine has to be stored in the refrigerator, according to the hospice nurses, because it regularly gets above seventy-seven degrees and at that temperature the medicine loses its potency or it becomes lethal or it will blow my grandfather up from the inside out, I DON'T KNOW I just do as I'm told.

On the kitchen counter next to the drying rack is a box of plastic syringes. They are thin and pencil-like, the kind you see zookeepers using to squirt formula into baby chipmunks' mouths to rehabilitate them before sending them back out into the world to fend for themselves.

The morphine is bright blue, the same lapis that electrocutes the underbelly of a glacier. Twice a day I am to fill the syringe to the intended line and shoot its contents into the back of my grandfather's throat. He is having difficulty swallowing these days, so the straighter shot I can get the better chance it has of being absorbed into his system. Sometimes I get ambitious and lean the syringe in a little too far and accidentally tap his uvula. He gags, I apologize and feel like a dick, which later makes me chuckle thinking about the number of oral swabs I've had to check for STIs after having God-knows-how-many dicks down my throat.

When you think of it this way, the syringe and the swabbing are something my grandfather and I have in common, though I don't tell him because (1) he wouldn't remember and (2) blowjobs aren't the kind of things you discuss with your dying grandfather despite his story being sandwiched in between many of them. Art, life, imitation.

Morphine tastes bitter, so it's best to wash it down with something. I didn't know this until one of the hospice nurses told me because I've never taken morphine and the stock in our refrigerator hasn't tempted me once. I doubt it would help with my kind of pain.

I fill up the syringe to its appropriate level and scoop a spoonful of chocolate cookie dough. I've been baking my sadness into sweets; this week alone I've adorned the kitchen counter with a peppermint cheesecake, two lemon loaves, and now chocolate cookies with white chips. I make my way to the ADA corridor. He stirs from his nap as I enter.

"How are you feeling, Grandpa?"

I sit on the edge of the bed and set my tools next to my thigh, out of view. I come in peace.

"I'm . . . alright." His voice sounds like tires pressed against gravel. He fiddles with the sheets for more than a moment. His fine motor skills are, well, less fine and less skilled. I relish that today he is moving. Gently, I pull the covers back.

"Are you hungry?"

His eyes are blank, and I know better than to ask again.

"I have medicine for you, will you open your mouth for me?"

"Medicine?" His brow would furrow if it could.

"Yes, it'll help you feel better. I promise."

"Well, alright."

He opens his mouth. I aim and shoot the liquid. He jerks his head to the side on impact. I imagine the chill is a shocking sensation, and the syringe nozzle is so skinny I wonder if the tiny stream feels sharp against his soft palate. He would not have the words to tell me if it does. I chase the morphine shot with a cookie-dough bite, and he swallows and relaxes. Almost immediately he closes his eyes and dozes back off. Morphine dribbles from my syringe onto the pillow, cerulean dots I dab with a tissue from his nightstand. I refill his water, turn off the lights, gather my spoon and syringe, and leave him be.

Upstairs I open the medicine cabinet in my bathroom. An orange bottle with a prescription stares back at me. We've done this routine every day since I filled it, and every day I shut the cabinet and push it out of my mind. Today I grab it and harvest one small pill from the canister.

ESTRADIOL. 2 mg. Take once a day with food.

It is also blue. It will also make things hurt less. I place it on my tongue, jackknife my head back, and swallow.

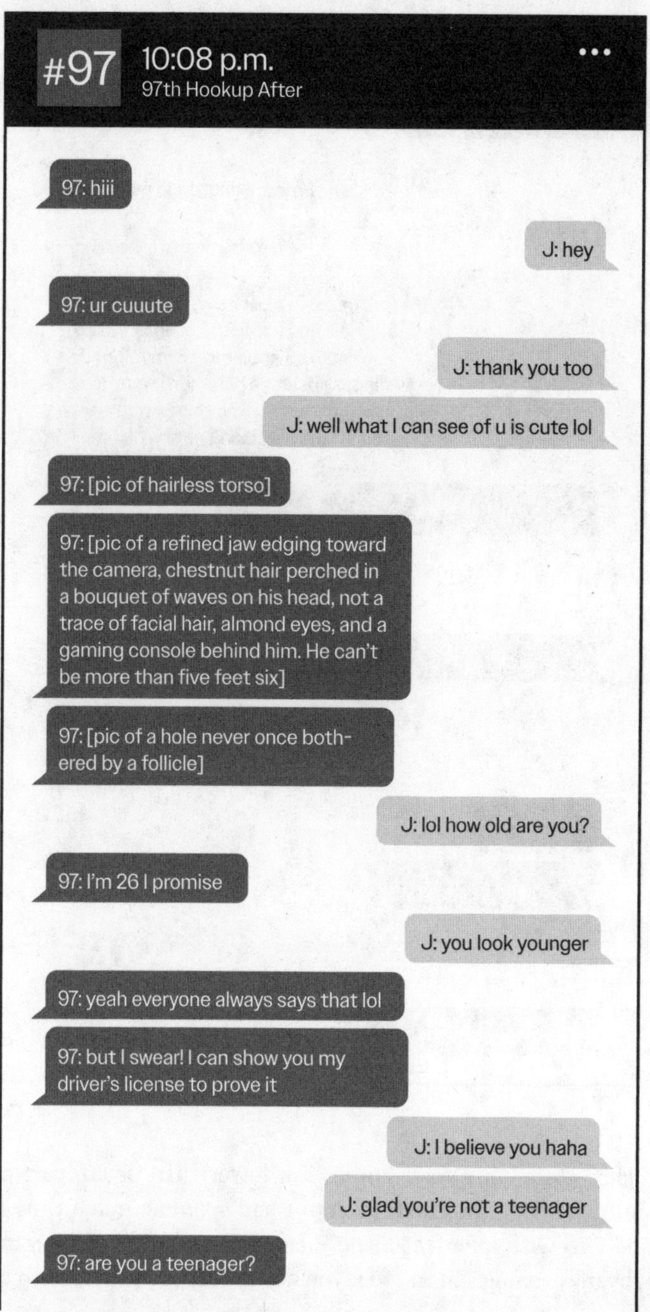
#97
10:08 p.m.
97th Hookup After
97: hiii
J: hey
97: ur cuuute
J: thank you too
J: well what I can see of u is cute lol
97: [pic of hairless torso]
97: [pic of a refined jaw edging toward the camera, chestnut hair perched in a bouquet of waves on his head, not a trace of facial hair, almond eyes, and a gaming console behind him. He can't be more than five feet six]
97: [pic of a hole never once both-ered by a follicle]
J: lol how old are you?
97: I'm 26 I promise
J: you look younger
97: yeah everyone always says that lol
97: but I swear! I can show you my driver's license to prove it
J: I believe you haha
J: glad you're not a teenager
97: are you a teenager?

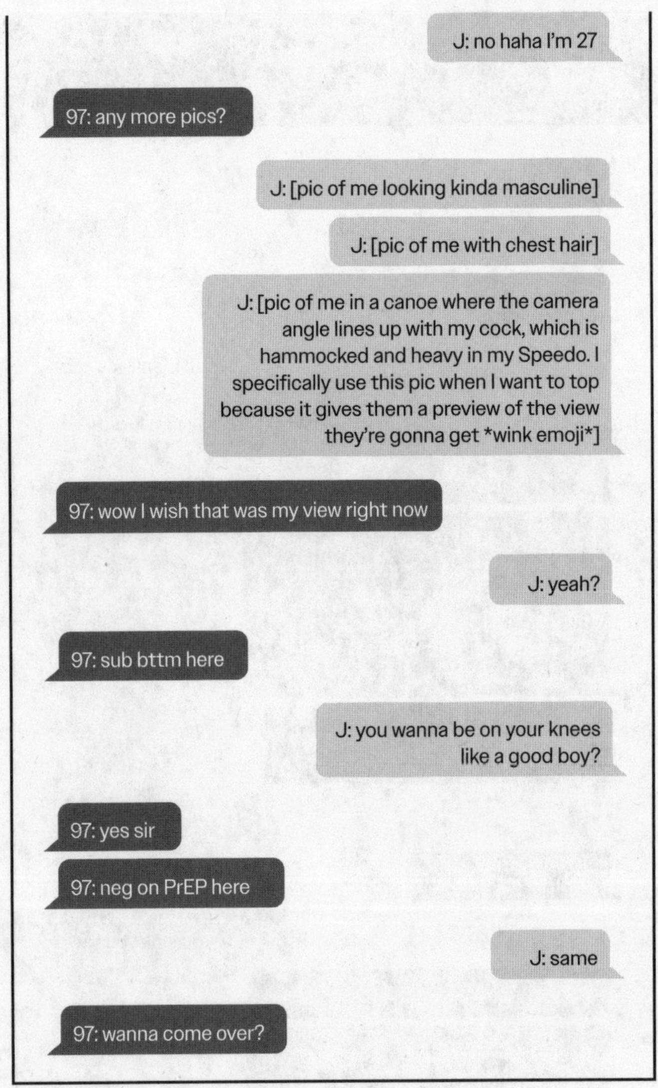

"Hey, cutie," my voice comes out lower than usual, part of the masculine affect I'd decided to don. I had spent so much time being a Good Girl with a Perfect Little Pussy (language collectively agreed upon by my evening suitors, so if you don't like it, take it up with them)

and I am curious if I still like being masculine in bed. I want to know if the fluidity of my gender carries into sexual energy too. I want to top. Here I am, little twink, get ready!

"Hi," he responds. He is tiny to the point where he has to push onto his tip toes to kiss me. He tastes like Listerine and lust and his tongue darts around mine playfully and he is the first boy that ever made me look like I had biceps by comparison. I am feeling masc and sexy! I am ready to be the top of his dreams!!! I feel my metaphorical backward hat cover me in boyish swagger. This must be how transmascs feel when they buy hoodies from Target and start saying things like "yo" and "I'm not really looking for a relationship right now." I secure my arms around his butt and lift him. He giggles and swings his legs around my back, hooking his ankles together. Now we're eye to eye.*

"You can put me wherever you want," he says, biting at my chest hair, which I haven't trimmed in at least a month because my grandfather has been dying and that wasn't a priority. I hope he likes it. The chest hair, not the dying. Out of the corner of my eyes I see the couch and hunker toward it, cute boy in tow. I squat and gently lay him down. He lets out a little moan, and his gym shorts bundle up toward his hips as his knees bend, ankles caught in my armpits. I release them and let him wiggle into the pillows. I know I have to make the next move, and I can tell he's waiting for it. Starting on top (especially as the top) comes with a fair bit of pressure; I set the pace! I set the tone! I decide what happens next! *Ahhhh!*

"Can I take this off, babe?" I curl my fingers around the base of his tank.

"Oh, yeah," he says, and I unsheathe his torso, discarding his shirt somewhere behind me. He does the same for me, and dives into the rest of my chest hair.

"These pecs, yum," he says, and I suppose at this angle and estrogen stage my breasts do, indeed, appear as pecs. I don't hate it. I go with it. I am cool and chill and masculine and about to be topping!! I lean

*If you find yourself getting to turned on at all of this please know I am not marketing this experience to you, rather allowing you into the inner workings of my sex life so you can understand this journey better. Think less about what I as a top can do for you in this moment and more about the literary picture I'm painting, hard as it may be. Ha! Get it? Hard? I digress.

forward and he assumes the same position: calves on my shoulders, body wedged among the couch cushions.

"Can I touch you here?" My hands are approaching his groin.

"Yeah, of course." His brow hints a furrow, but it dissipates into our next kiss. I'm rolling my palm around his junk like a stick shift and feeling it upgrade gears in real time.

"Can I put my hands under your shorts?" I breathe. His hands have latched themselves to my stubble, and he holds my face at arm's distance.

"I told you, you can do whatever you want to me. You don't have to ask. I'm your good boy, remember?"

"I just wanted to make sure!"

He ignores my defense, hops off the couch and onto his knees.

"May I?" He looks up coyly.

"Yes, please." I place my hands on the back of his head like a Sean Cody model as he pulls the rest of my clothes to the carpet and fixes his lips to the hardest part of me. I am surprised to be so erect; I had anticipated a decrease in functionality with the estrogen. It seems not to have reached my cock and perhaps stopped at my chest. I don't mind. In fact I like it, and judging by the sounds I'm hearing from the boy on his knees, so does he.

I lift him by the chin to kiss him, which was my way of politely ending the adequate (but not extraordinary) blowjob I'd just received, and say, "Do you want me to fuck you?"

"Yes sir!"

Sir.

I start him on the couch, he begs me to pin his hands back. I let him ride me, he finds the most pleasure when I hold his hips in place and jackhammer from underneath. This isn't particularly sustainable, so I pick him up, maintaining our connection (hot, I know, I've been working on this trick for years) and drill him into the wall. He squeals things like, "Ooh god," and, "Fuck me, sir," and whatever else they're saying on TimTales these days. We end up on the carpet on all fours. I prop a leg up and pull at his hips. He arches, moans, melts, repeats.

Suddenly I am terrified I am a rapist.

I didn't ask to flip him into doggy. We just . . . kinda did it. He turned, or I turned him? He might've said *Put it in me,* but I don't remember. I am all too unsure if we hit the crossroads of Rape or Not

Rape and while I understand this is an irrational fear given the muffled chorus of *thank you* and *fuck yeah* and *harder, sir* coming from where his nose is slotted between the couch cushions, I can't curb it. The fear flushes the blood from my dick and I have to pull out and regroup.

"You ok? Shit, did I have an accident?"

"No! You're great." I pat his butt, stroking myself, willing my dick to harden again so we can finish. It flops against my palm like a fish.

"Sometimes he just needs a break." I drop the fish, letting it dangle. "It's not you, I promise!"

"Well, this feels amazing"—he squeezes the fish—"and it was really hot the way you were using my ass."

I exhale at the affirmative and cover it by pretending to catch my breath.

"Yeah." I search for something to say. "You felt great too."

He wags his invisible tail. "Thanks, daddy."

Can trans femmes be daddies? I don't hate it, but I don't necessarily like it either. Maybe it's fine? My gender, my rules, right?

"Do you want me to get you off?" I ask.

His fish is flopped like mine. This often happens to bottoms, especially submissive bottoms, whose lack of erection is often attributed to the overwhelm of pleasurable sensations they're feeling other places. It still feels polite to offer.

"Oh, I'm good. I do want you to fuck me again, though." He bends down as if he is going to take the fish in his mouth, an idea that makes me want to shrivel.

"Could we, um, could we cuddle instead for a minute?"

He cocks his head, as if the proposition was unusual. "Sure."

He springs up, rearranging the cushions, and I lie down with a heave. He climbs into the remaining couch space, chestnut hair tickling my ears, fingers drawing swirls in my chest hair. He wriggles.

"What?" I tease.

"I wanted to get closer to you!" He wriggles again. It's charming. In a burst of energy I turn to my side and pull him into me, engulfing my little spoon into a fort built out of my limbs. He giggles and sends a line of kisses up my forearm. I secure my hand between his chest and his armpit. Going for the boob. I push that out of my mind. I'm rushed with the desire to kiss this retriever puppy of a boy and squeeze him in all the right spots. I want to make sure he is adored and cared for and played with and fucked and not abandoned, and while cognitively I realize I don't know anything about this guy, I'm pulling this soliloquy of desires out of wherever it's lay barren in the bowels of my brain, I feel how I feel. Maybe I'm just relieved that I'm not a rapist.

I wonder if I actually want him to feel those things or if I'm putting these thoughts into the universe as some kind of karmic correction for whatever Finnegan is doing out there. Or maybe I'm doing it so I know it's possible, to give myself hope that if I'm capable of it, after all of this and everything, which means that someone else, one day, will be able to do it for me.

He rolls over with a throaty purr. The trans girl inside me wonders if I should turn over and let him spoon me. Just for a moment.

He's cute, but that isn't enough. My surge of cute aggression has dissipated, and soon he's going to use whatever tricks are up his sleeve to get me back in the mood and back inside him. The idea of fucking him again is unfathomable. I know I'm not a rapist, but the fact that I have the power to take it that far frightens me. It strikes me as odd that I only feel this fear when I'm topping, and then I think deeper and decide it makes sense. Often to penetrate is to hold power, and rape is about power. To receive is to trust the other person with that power. There is so much trust required in sex and I'm not sure I trust my body yet. The signals are too strong, too inconsistent, too heavily influenced by triggers my brain hasn't learned to file properly. Despite having nearly a hundred men after my rapist I am still, in more ways than I know, at war with my own body. I want to trust it. I want to trust the men I sleep with. I want to allow myself to transition in peace. I want a break. I don't want this boy anymore, and I don't want to be on this couch.

"You're such a sexy man." He runs his fingers through my chest hair with a tug. I wince. "Never shave this, please."

I buzz it off as soon as I get home.

Finn, After

A series of texts I wish my then-boyfriend Finnegan sent me in the days after I was raped when I was bedridden:

October 28:

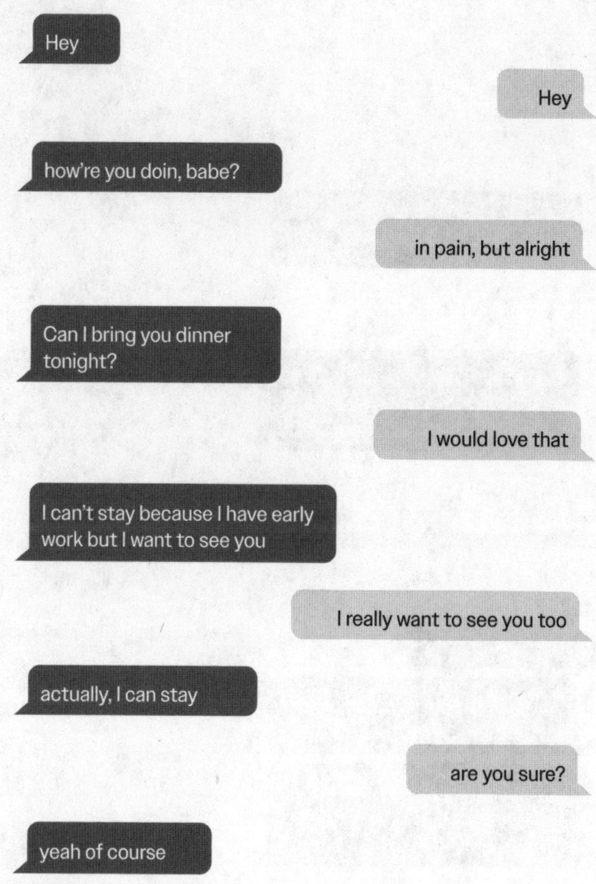

October 30:

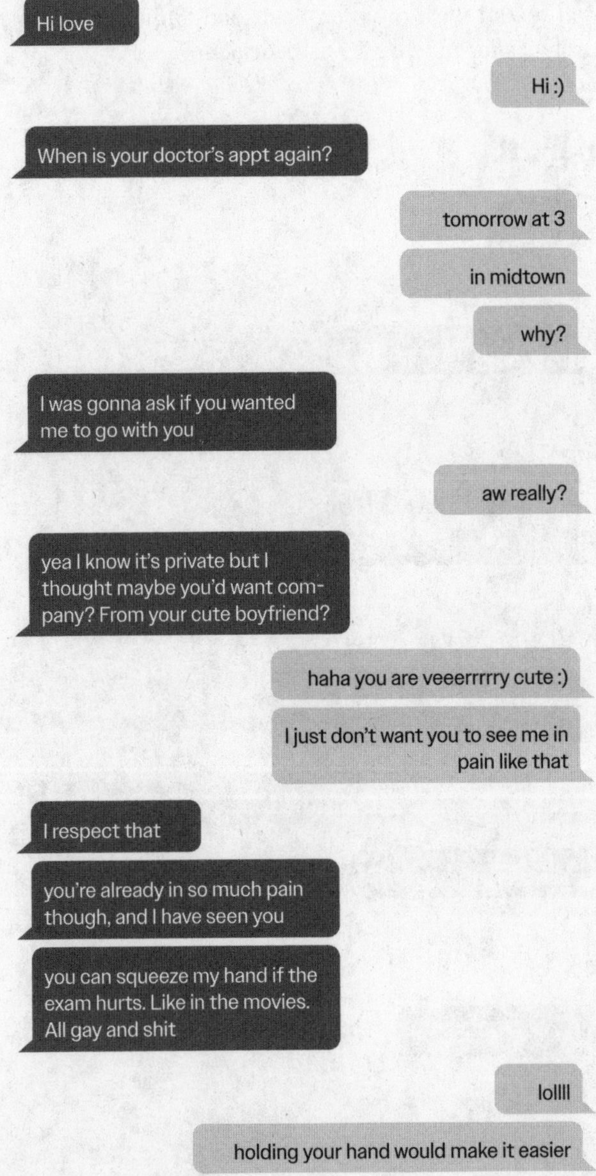
Hi love
Hi :)
When is your doctor's appt again?
tomorrow at 3
in midtown
why?
I was gonna ask if you wanted me to go with you
aw really?
yea I know it's private but I thought maybe you'd want company? From your cute boyfriend?
haha you are veeerrrrry cute :)
I just don't want you to see me in pain like that
I respect that
you're already in so much pain though, and I have seen you
you can squeeze my hand if the exam hurts. Like in the movies. All gay and shit
lollll
holding your hand would make it easier

I'm gonna uber there, do you wanna meet me up here or down there?

I'll be coming from work so can I meet you there?

ok perf

thank you. that really means so much to me that you would come

of course babe. I want to help.

November 1:

this is a reminder that I think you're beautiful and I want to be with you and we are gonna get through this together

I love you

I love you too

November 2:

hey, FaceTime you in 10? I'm on a break

ok!

November 3:

So i'm thinking of posting about this on IG

yeah?

yeah idk it just feels right

like with the me too movement and stuff

it just feels weird to be silent, and i'm gonna have to tell everyone at work anyway since I can't move that well

if you feel it's the right thing I support you

do you not think it's the right thing?

no I do! It's super brave

I can't imagine telling everyone something like that

but you've always been transparent with everything and i think it's amazing

you should do it

thanks what do you think of this caption

[sends caption]

wow that's . . . that's really rough, but it's important.

i don't really know how to respond

your heart is so big

i'm in awe of you

awwww babe

i'm serious

thank you

i can't wait to be in your arms again

tomorrow! I'll hold you all night

[This is the part where Finn and I have sex for the first time after I was raped, and I still cry, except instead of looking me in the eyes and saying, *I knew you would cry,* he stops and says, *We don't have to keep going, are you ok?* and I say, *Yes, I'm just really emotional about this and I want you to feel pleasure and I'm afraid I'm not giving it to you,* and he lands on the pillow next to me and says, *Sweetheart, this isn't about me right now, this is about you. Let's take a break,* so we cuddle and I cry a few more times on and off because I am happy and lucky and healing and not at all abandoned.]

November 6:

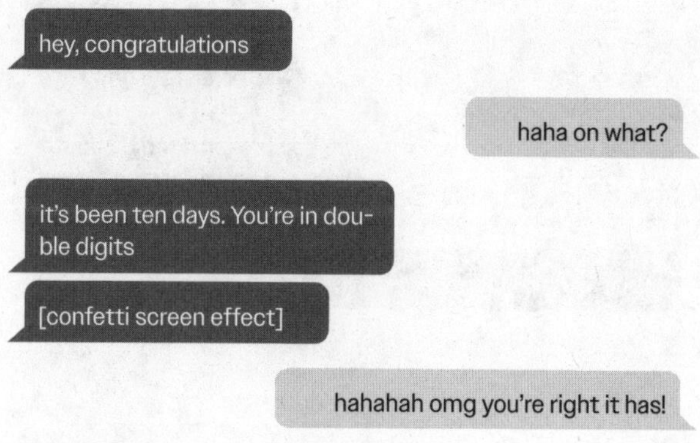

November 11:

was thinking about you at work

was thinking about you as I lay here in this bed with my broken asshole!!

jesus christ

no its funny you can laugh

ok can i say a joke

PLEASE DO

I wish it was me who broke your asshole

wink

NOT IN A RAPEY WAY

in a like, we had really good sex way

omfg hahahahah

that was honestly a good one

I wish you had broken it too bc then it might not actually be so broken

are u saying my peepee is smol

NO OMG

I'M SAYING YOU WOULDN'T HAVE HURT ME LIKE THAT

unless I wanted it ;)

we've never had rough sex before

would you be . . . into that?

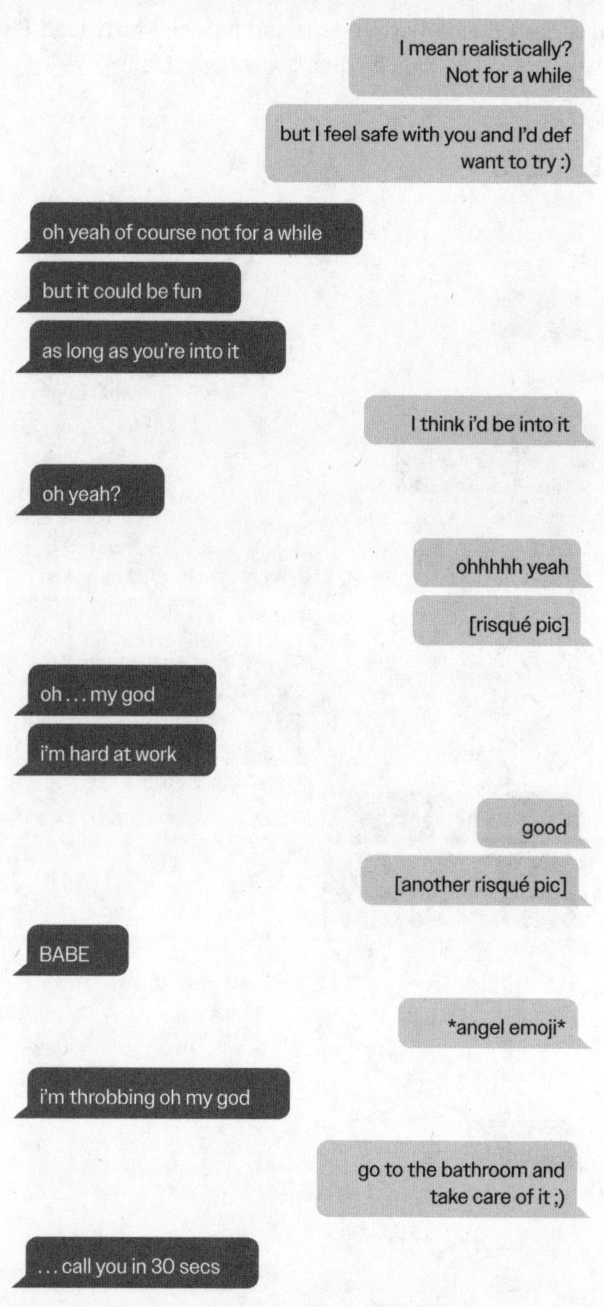
I mean realistically?
Not for a while
but I feel safe with you and I'd def want to try :)
oh yeah of course not for a while
but it could be fun
as long as you're into it
I think i'd be into it
oh yeah?
ohhhhh yeah
[risqué pic]
oh . . . my god
i'm hard at work
good
[another risqué pic]
BABE
angel emoji
i'm throbbing oh my god
go to the bathroom and take care of it ;)
. . . call you in 30 secs

The real series of texts between me and my then-boyfriend Finnegan in the days after I was raped when I was bedridden:

October 29:

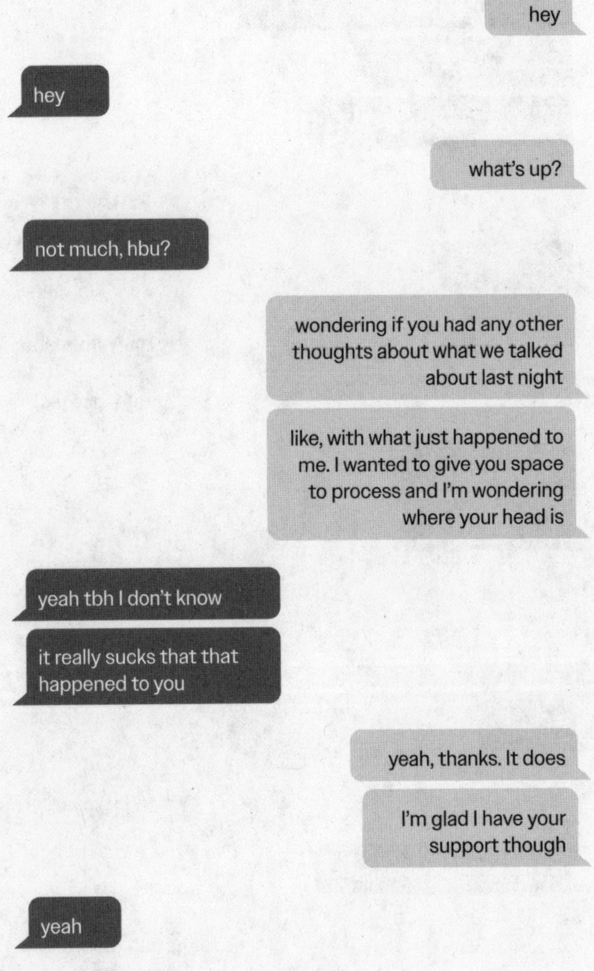

October 30:

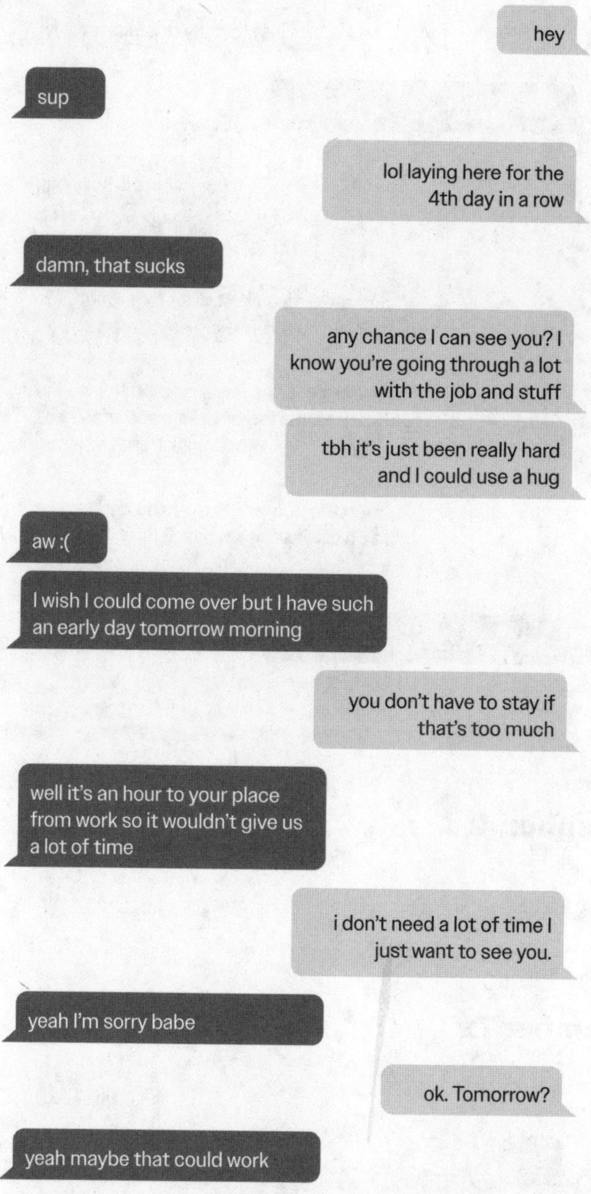
hey
sup
lol laying here for the 4th day in a row
damn, that sucks
any chance I can see you? I know you're going through a lot with the job and stuff
tbh it's just been really hard and I could use a hug
aw :(
I wish I could come over but I have such an early day tomorrow morning
you don't have to stay if that's too much
well it's an hour to your place from work so it wouldn't give us a lot of time
i don't need a lot of time I just want to see you.
yeah I'm sorry babe
ok. Tomorrow?
yeah maybe that could work

November 1:

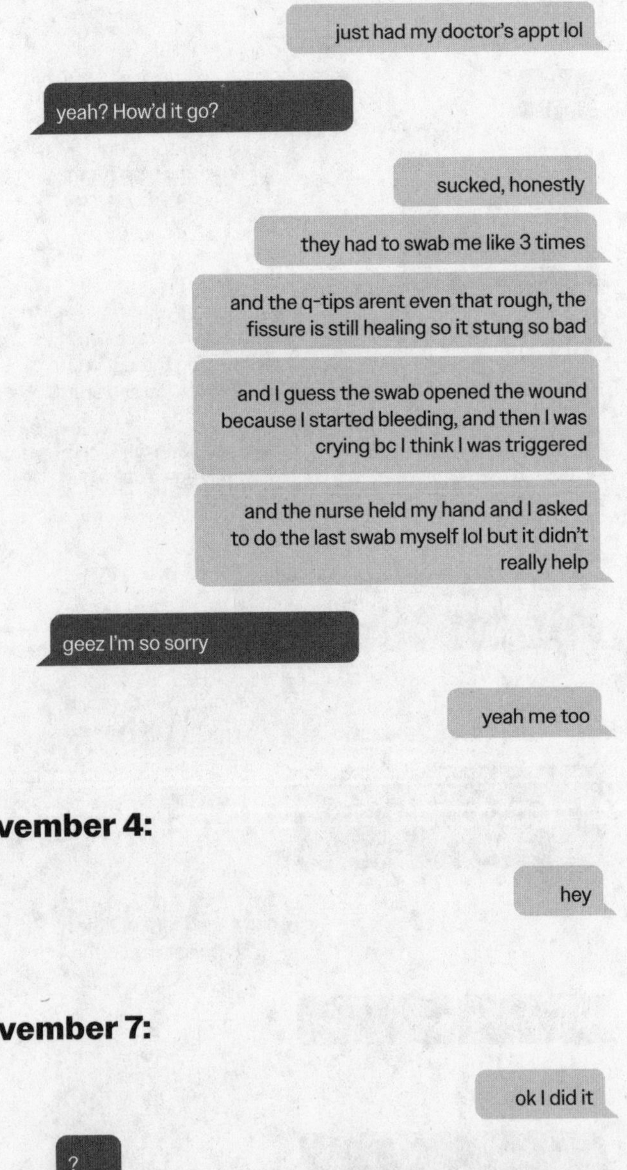

November 4:

November 7:

posted on insta! Like we talked about!

oh good!

like kinda nervous but idk i think it's the right thing to do?

yeah for sure

and I changed a couple things in the caption but I still think it gets the message across?

it does!

you read it?

reading it now

oh hehe

it's good!

yeah? You think so?

yeah its really beautiful

I already got a DM from someone I know who had a similar experience. A guy, actually. A dancer

damn, what did he say?

that he had a similar experience and he thought he was the only one. said he's sorry it happened to me but thinks it's brave of me for posting and rly necessary

aw that's really sweet

yeah

just got another

another DM?

yeah, someone I went to middle school with, actually. Says she went through the same thing and she couldn't tell anyone and was so alone

she sent me her # too in case I needed to talk

I literally haven't talked to her in ten years

like, wow I'm kinda floored by that

yeah damn that's crazy

ok another one, another guy who was like "I'm so glad you're speaking up on this because I know 3 other guys who have stories like yours. I'm sorry this happened and pls reach out if you need anything."

it's just wild how many people I know that have stories like this?

and it's wild how many boys are in your DMs now lol

that's . . . not the point?

no I know it was just funny

this is really important to me. I was really scared to share this.

and people are liking it! It has over a hundred likes in ten minutes! That's good!

it's not about the likes

It's about how many other people I know who have also been sexually assaulted

no one is talking about this but apparently it's happening often

November 9:

hey, I thought it was kinda odd that you never responded to me the other day—what happened?

nothing I got distracted at work. Sorry, I should've responded

thanks.

am I gonna get to see you? It's been ten days.

I miss you.

I miss you too! I'll see you soon.

when?

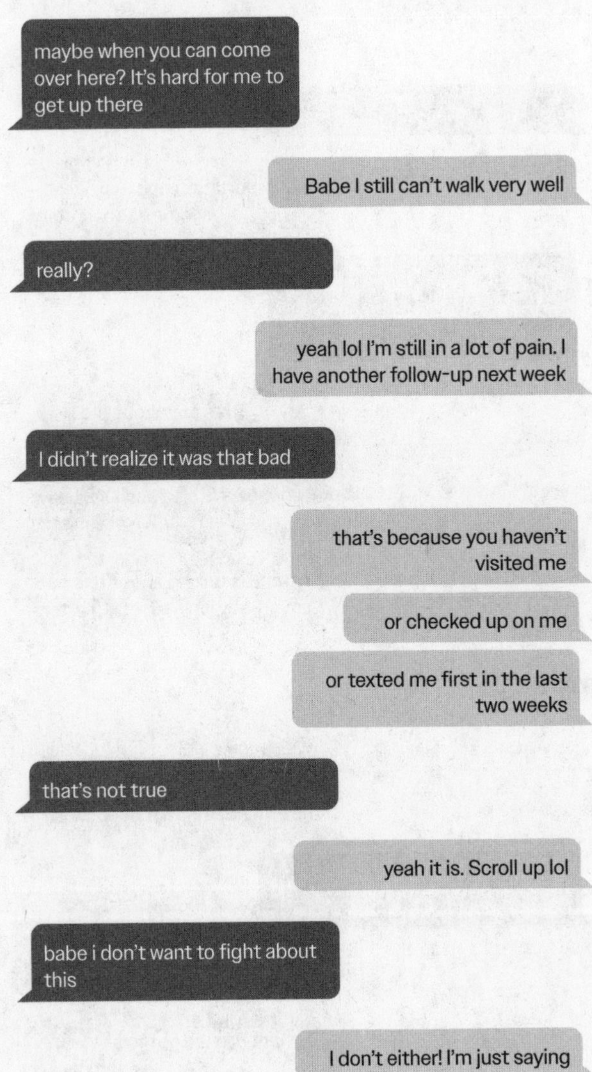

[This is the part where Finn and I text all flirty and I go over to his place despite being in pain and we do, somehow, have sex and I cry and he says, *I just knew you were gonna cry* and the part I didn't tell you was that after we finished he sent me home because he had to work early or just *wanted alone time*.]

hey, i'm really glad I got to see you last night

me too babe

Can I see you again this week? It really helps me when I do

yeah, sunday?

Sunday, November 11:

hey

?

Tuesday, November 13:

hey, I think we need to talk.

I am separating the granola from the roasting pan with a spatula when my grandfather is wheeled around the corner by my grandmother, with some effort. He is swaddled in blankets, for he is perpetually cold these days, despite it being an unseasonably warm March. His head bobs as they round a curve.

"Good morning!"

I plunge a spoon into the vat of Greek yogurt and deposit three spoonfuls into as many bowls. I repeat with a second serving. He says nothing.

"Would you like some yogurt?"

He aspirates, as if to speak, but the effort is in vain. It sounds like cracked wind escaping from his throat. My grandmother parks him by the kitchen table and offers him water.

"Well, if you're hungry, I have some yogurt with granola." I place the bowl and accompanying spoon in front of him. He looks at it with what appears to be astonishment. He reaches his left hand out and grabs the bowl by its lip, fingers smushed into the food. He is about to lift it when my grandmother catches it, wrangles it from his grip, and passes it to me behind his wheelchair, out of sight. He gazes off toward something we cannot see. He spends no more than two more minutes at the table before managing to say the word "tired." My grandmother wheels him back to his room. I set the empty pan under the running faucet. That's all we see of him today.

Finn, After

I don't remember much about the breakup. I do remember that he was two hours late. I remember because I sat in the Whole Foods above Bryant Park on the phone with my mom half sorting out why I was still there waiting and half passing the time. He was visiting a friend, one from college. He had refused to commit to a time because he "didn't know how long it would take" since he "hadn't seen her in so long." I asked if it was possible to set a cutoff time since I was in pain, and it would take a lot of effort to get to midtown but of course you can infer his value system at this point.

When he finally did arrive, I had moved to a corner table in the park. He set down his backpack. No kiss, no hug, no "how are you?" Just sat there.

I don't know who spoke first. It was probably me. I remember the green metal of the park chairs and I remember hooking my foot underneath one of the legs. I remember facing away from him on a diagonal. I don't remember seeing his eyes, and if I did they weren't oceans. I probably said something about how it hurt that he didn't visit me or reach out, that after I posted about the rape on Instagram people came out of the woodwork to support me but my own boyfriend never even so much as called.

I vaguely recall his saying something to the tune of "I didn't know how to take care of you. I didn't know how to fix it."

And I vaguely recall saying, "I never asked you to fix it. I just wanted to know you at least cared about me enough to walk six blocks and that we'd get through this together."

I think he said he was "going through a lot," and I looked at him dumbfounded because of the two of us, only one of us had an anal fissure that might require surgery as a byproduct of being sexually assaulted fourteen days ago, and I wasn't really sure how his "a lot" trumped that exactly.

I know I said, "I'm going through a lot too, Finn."

And he said, "I'm just not ready for this."

"For what?"

"For . . ." He trailed off.

"For a relationship?"

"Well, maybe." He studied his shoes. "It's not about you. I just don't know that I'm cut out to be in a relationship right now."

"Finn, you are absolutely cut out to be in a relationship. That's what we've been doing for the last six months. I get that this is a hurdle—believe me, I get it—but we can work through this. I mean, we love each other, so I want to work through this. Don't you?"

He was silent, seemingly fascinated by his laces. I was losing to a pair of shoes.

"Don't you?"

"I DON'T KNOW!" It was the first time I'd ever heard him yell. "I just . . . I don't feel the way I should."

"About what?"

"About . . ."

I knew what he was going to say, but I refused to finish the sentence for him. I wanted to hear him say it. He didn't. Instead, he said:

"It's, well, a lot has changed since I came back from Japan. You've changed, I've changed, and I've been enjoying the fact that our relationship is open—"

"Oh, you've been seeing Arnie?"

"Please don't bring him into th—"

"I'm not the one who brought him into anything. It just seems like a strange time to bring up how much you're enjoying fucking other people considering I couldn't have sex if I wanted to."

Exasperation sucked the air from Finn's teeth. "My point is it's making me realize that I don't think a relationship is the right decision for me right now, I guess."

I grasped for a singular logical thread toward the conclusion that abandoning me after everything I'd been through was the right course of action. My temper trembled. He couldn't even bring himself to say, "I don't want to be with you." He had decided on "a relationship isn't right for me." Maybe in his head it was the most gentle way to let me down, but once spoken it made him sound a coward. He looked five years old, eyes glued to his high-tops. I wanted to slap him or shake him or yell or something to rattle the words "What am I saying? I don't want to break up!" out of him so we could go back to my apartment and kiss and make up and be alright. Of course, he did no such thing, and neither did I.

"So . . . you want to break up?" My voice was steel.

"I'm sorry."

I stared at him. "Really? Really, Finnegan?" For the first time he met my gaze.

"James, it's . . you're not the confident person I fell in love with anymore."

The words slit a fissure clean down my heart. He kept going.

"I'm sorry, but you're not. You're not the confident person I fell in love with. That person was fiery and passionate and wouldn't let anything knock them down! You were funny and always willing to make a joke and never took anything too seriously. You didn't need constant attention or validation because you took pride in your independence and now suddenly all of that is gone? The person I love, the person I want to marry one day is just . . . gone?"

"Finn." My voice was small. "There's a reason for that—"

"I know! You've had a rough time! But when am I going to get James back?"

"I don't know, I'm trying to heal but this takes time and it's been two wee—"

"Two weeks!!!" he cut me off. "Two weeks and you're not making any progress!"

"I'm sorry, am I on a fucking clock here? I was raped, Finnegan. A man split open my insides because he wouldn't take no for an answer, and now I can barely walk, I can't work, I might have to have a surgery that costs ten thousand dollars, and I can't even get ahold of my boyfriend to meet me and even talk about all of this, and it turns out you're just biding your time waiting for me to be confident again?"

I was crying, which only made me angrier.

"Do you know how this works? When someone rapes you, when someone violates you in this way, they take the most vulnerable part of your spirit and they break it. My spirit is broken, Finn, and I'm not asking you to fix it. I know you can't, and it would be unfair to ask. What I'm asking is for you to stick by me and tell me you love me and that we'll get through this. That's all I'm asking. Can you do that?"

He almost looked at his shoes.

"Don't look at your fucking shoes, look me in the eyes." What was left of the oceans was still. "Can you do that?"

You know the answer now as well as I did then. He couldn't. He got up, mumbled an apology, and slung his backpack over his shoulder. My asshole throbbed from sitting on the green metal park chair.

The confident person he fell in love with watched his Abercrombie shoulders vanish onto Sixth Avenue, taking her partner, her friend, her future marriage, every laugh, and every I love you in the backpack he carried, leaving her with the gruesome knowledge that if she just could figure out a way to be herself again, if she just wasn't broken, if she just hadn't been raped, he wouldn't be leaving. He'd be off to work or to see a friend or wherever and he'd be back that night to hold her and kiss her and fuck her and wake up next to her.

But he wouldn't do that, he'd go find someone else who hadn't been raped fourteen days prior to hold and kiss and fuck and love and wake up next to and marry. He was leaving her, disappearing into the latticework of New Yorkers crossing the street, and it was all her fault.

I stand at the precipice of the ADA hallway, just before the wood turns to carpet. I'm listening for a sign that he's awake. The sheets rustle, and then again. It's almost time for his morphine. My grandmother is asleep upstairs, so I'll administer this dose. Rustling again. I decide to enter.

"Hi," I say softly. He tries to vocalize, or he grunts, I'm not sure. He looks so peaceful, white hair combed to the side, blankets packed tightly, arms barely peeking out. The sun slices through the blinds. We can hear the red birds, his favorite. I am sure he can hear them because it almost looks like he's smiling.

I climb onto the bed, careful not to jostle him, and lie down so we are face-to-face. His eyes are open.

"Hello," I say softer. "It's me, James."

He nods. I am embarrassed that I'm relieved, but I am. I remain one of the only family members this disease hasn't spooned out of his mind. I remain by his side. We remain together.

The fan whirrs, its metal chain swinging limply in oblong circles over our heads. His palm is open on his pillow. I fit my hand inside his. It is leathery, warm, the same size as mine.

"I love you." I tell him with the urgency of knowing how few chances I have left to say this. The words come slow, like the last remaining drops from a closed faucet.

He draws in a breath, and I wonder if he is about to say something. He doesn't, or he can't. His breath is rank, metallic. I remember the morphine and I begin to sit up. His grip on my hand stops me. I lie back down.

His white hair stirs under the fan and I think about what it means to have lived eighty years on this planet. I wonder if I'll make it to eighty before I have to hold a Funeral Pregame because I've fallen to the same fate as him. His grip reminds me of the infamous infant death grip. It makes me wonder if Alzheimer's is paring back his memories and movements in reverse chronology. Maybe this regression is stripping him age by age, year by year, memory by memory, and when it reaches inception he will die. Embryo must be close now.

"Do you remember how you used to take me to Barnes and Noble every time I would visit you?" He doesn't answer, but if he can hear me at all, I want him to hear this story.

"When I was nine or ten, I loved *A Wrinkle in Time*, and I asked if we could get the sequel. You told me my cousins loved *Harry Potter*, and you asked if I wanted one of those books as well, but I said I didn't think that woman was a good writer like Madeleine L'Engle. What's funny is the woman who wrote *Harry Potter* turned into a horrible person, so I'd like to think I always had exceptional taste. Anyway, you laughed and bought me the sequel and a few other books. We sat at the café table eating one of those big chocolate chip cookies and discussing which books we thought were best; acclaimed writers, Newbery Medal winners, something I pulled from Oprah's book club that I'm sure you deemed inappropriate for me."

Once upon a time he might've laughed. Now he just stares. He keeps my hand in his. I keep going.

"The other day I went looking for that book, the sequel, and I couldn't find it. I was sure I kept it here, but for all I know it's at my parents' house, or we gave it away, I don't know. I guess it doesn't really matter though, because you gave me the love of reading, and books, and literature and I will always be grateful for that."

His eyes are wide, intent, awake. I hope more than anything he can hear what I'm saying. I don't know how many chances I have left to say this. I don't know how many more days he'll be awake.

"Thank you for taking me to the bookstore every year when I was growing up. I think I will look for you in every bookstore forever when you're gone. Maybe I'll even write a book one day, who knows."

He blinks. The corner of his mouth softens. One of my tears tumbles down my cheekbone and lands on the pillow. I am not embarrassed. I let it be.

"We are going to miss you so much," I say, and then think maybe that's an awful, inconsiderate thing to say to someone on the precipice of death who might be terrified of leaving their family behind for grief's crevasse to swallow them. I try again. "Grandpa, if it's your time, I understand. I will let you go. And I will be ok."

I think I see him smile, but it is too fast for me to catch. A flicker of crimson lands just out of view. I lift my head and see three red birds on the windowsill, little brown feet clustered into the shade, silent, watching as the comforter rises and falls with his breath.

Finn, Before

The night lights of Manhattan speckled the window behind Finn's head. We shared a pillow, nose to nose, his arm around me while I traced the line of his bicep with my fingerprints. He was leaving tomorrow, for the other side of the globe, for work. I couldn't think about it. I fastened my brain to this moment: Be here, be now. Memorize the architecture of his arm hair thinning above his elbow, the angle of his nose as it slopes. Remember the exact shade of his lips, the way the pigment blooms in dusty pinks across his mouth. Capture the sensation of his legs interlaced with yours, hip to hip, cock to cock, belly to belly. Notice the way the covers sink into the saddle between his rib cage and his pelvis. See him here, now, with you. The memory will stay, even if he can't.

"I'm sorry I keep crying during sex," I said, hiding the next tear by smushing my cheek into the pillow.

"I saw that." He giggled and kissed my nose.

"It's just because . . . I feel safe with you."

His eyes shifted, melty glaciers rearranging, cutting new territory, widening, softening, breathing me into swirls of cerulean. I watched the whole world unfold around his pupils, a world where I could dive into their blue warmth and be held forever.

"I love you," he said for the first time.

"I love you too."

Dive, swirl, plummet.

I fell asleep in his arms.

If you're ever in Manhattan and you take the C to Chambers Street and follow the signs to exit on the last staircase before the end of the platform, when you emerge from the underground transit system you'll be at the 9/11 memorial.

The giant swirling memorial bottom pools will be on your right, the oculus on your left, and just past it will be a building called 175 Greenwich. If you manage to get past security, head to the tenth floor and you'll find the coworking space I paid an exorbitant amount of money for to write part of this book. And if you're there late, you might find a man from a tech start-up who has the east window in his office, and you can softly knock on his door and say *I know this sounds so silly but can I see the view from your office?* and he'll look at you sort of funny but say *alright* (probably because you are beautiful and he is an ally to the trans community) and from his floor-to-ceiling window you can look straight down onto the pool that commemorates the South Tower, the first to fall. And instead of wanting to dive into the slippery, slate-gray, city-block-size drain and escape everything, you will be struck by how small it looks.

People dart around it like pearls spilled from a broken necklace and taxis skid before crosswalks and peanut vendors populate the perimeter and you will see so much life dotted around on the ground that your brow will furrow because there is a whole world buzzing amidst the memory of doom and tragedy. In fact, there are more trees than you can count, green as emeralds, pushing from the curbsides to the pool's edges. You'll look back at the slate gray only to find it has turned silver, and you'll look to the plummeting hole only to have it obscured by the city's brightness; sonorous beams from TVs tucked inside two-bedroom apartments and filmy fluorescents from end-of-work-day office spaces and dampened yellows from pizza parlor windows and blood-red brake signals from bumbling Lyft drivers and the never-ending streams of light, light, light.

And even you will be light, light, light,

lighter.

And I can't tell you that you won't hate Mr. Anderson or your rapist anymore,

And I don't think it will make terrorism or sexual violence any easier to handle,

But you will see more life than death and maybe the fragments of hatred and hurt will unstitch and fall like debris onto the street below.

You might think of your rapist bustling about his own city and wonder if he has anyone to go home to, if he ever thinks of you, whether you'll ever see him again, whether his heart is also broken.

And you might cry and if you do I hope the trans ally pats your shoulder or gets you a tea from the kitchen you're both paying too much money to use.

And you will end your membership at the coworking space where you look at 9/11 every day because you won't need it anymore.

You've seen enough.

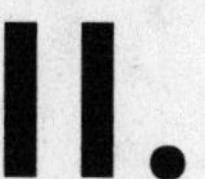

Everyone thinks it's a terrible idea, but I've decided to visit my rapist. I am afraid he doesn't know the severity of what he did to me. I'm afraid that he is raping other people and he doesn't know. I'm afraid he's doing well. I'm afraid I cannot hold the politic of restorative justice unless I practice it. I am afraid I am still attracted to him. I'm afraid of forgiving him. I'm afraid I can't forgive him. I'm afraid he will remember me. I'm afraid he won't. I'm afraid of him. I'm afraid of myself around him. I think the only way to overcome the fear is to go through it, and the only way I maintain a modicum of control is by visiting him in a public place. Somewhere it would be difficult to rape me. Again. I want our first interaction since the incident to be one I've prepared for. I don't want to be worried about running into him on the street. I don't want to keep running into his memory when other men touch me. I want control. I want to get this over with. I want to move on.

I rent a car. It's a 2022 Kia Soul. It looks like a toaster. I drive to his city. Hours later I pull into the parking lot. Neon signs flash SOULCYCLE. I put the car in park. Through the latticework windows I see him immediately: black shirt, black shorts, headset balanced in his ears. The left ear is one-eighth of an inch higher than the right. He adjusts the headset and smiles at a ponytail with purple leggings. They hug. I hate her because he's nice to her. His biceps bubble at the elbow, just enough to say, "I lift less than I cycle," but "One time I held down this hot nonbinary girl and didn't listen to her when she said no." Ponytail says something. His eyes crinkle, he laughs, she enters the studio.

I pull the key from the ignition. It snags on the windshield-wiper control. The windshield wipers begin frantically squeaking across the dash. It startles me. I turn them off. I place the keys in my pocket. I am afraid Ponytail looks better in her leggings than I do in mine. Hers scream "fun at parties" and mine scream "victim." I check myself out in the latticework windows. My "victim" still looks fantastic. I tell myself I will not kill myself, no matter what he says or what happens. I will survive this. I will survive him. I am in control. I trust my body. I can do this.

"Heeeyyy, welcome!" The door swings open. The left arm that once pinned down my shoulder now holds the door open for me. The SoulCycle emblem printed on the sleeve stares back at me: a skull and crossbones.

I slip past. I'm taller than he is. I had forgotten this, or I didn't know it because we didn't spend much time standing. He's the kind of blond where his eyelashes are thick and invisible at the same time. His left incisor is capped with tiny ridges that look like the letter *m* on repeat. I'm meeting my other half, again. The other half of every therapy session, every nightmare, every tear-stricken moment of attempted intimacy with a man for the last five years. He's gorgeous. I wonder if he really is the same person.

"I don't think I've met you before." A sly grin uncovers the incisor. "Have I?"

He doesn't know me. I'm safe. It must be the long hair or the estrogen or the fact that he barely looked at my face because he was too busy getting what he wanted. I flash a smile in return.

"I don't think I've met you either." I pause for effect. "But I'm verrrryyyy glad we've met now."

"Oh yeah?" His eyes flick to my beltline and back up. Instantly I am comfortable because now I have power. He wants me, which makes me just as rape-able as the first time we met, though perhaps slightly more human.

A voice from behind the desk cuts the tension. “I can check in whoever’s next!”

I offer her the fake name I registered under, hoping she won’t request a license for verification. She doesn’t. Instead, she hands me a clipboard with a liability waiver. Years ago, I all but signed one when I messaged him back:

Ok great, be there in ten!

“Well,” he leans against the front desk, shakes his hair, and smooths it over with fingers that once felt like screws. “I guess I’ll see you after class?”

“I guess you will.” I return the clipboard, and leave him with the echo of my cooing in his ears.

I pick a bike toward the back of the studio. He mounts the instructor bike in the center like a swordsman mounting a horse before battle. He serenades the room of Lululemon-wrapped soccer moms with his cheesy, “take it at your own pace” facade buttoned with “ARE YOU READY TO SWEAT?”

I am. He doesn’t know it, but when I tell him why I’m here he’ll be sweating too.

***

Because he is the rock star that somehow made fifty-five minutes on a bike that goes nowhere feel like a dance party, there is a line to talk to him in the lobby after class. I hover toward the back as Lululemon Mom #1 drags on about her gay son (he’s in fourth grade, she knows he’s gay even though he hasn’t said so, and even better, thinks it’s appropriate to tell her spin instructor!), followed by Lululemon Mom #2 whose divorce is taking longer than expected and she really needed this today, and Ponytail (fuck her, I don’t know what she said and I don’t care, those are definitely extensions) all say their piece. Finally, the front desk lobby is clear.

“Well, look who stuck around!” He claps his palms in front of him.

“Yeah, I did.” I’m not flirting anymore.

“So . . . what did you think?”

"I think we need to talk."

"What?"

I glance around, aware the person behind the front desk can hear everything we're saying even from halfway across the room.

"I'm not even here!" She chirps, moving toward the studio. "I have to go clean the bikes anyway!"

The door closes behind her and he looks at me with concern. It startles me because it is the first time he has ever looked at me with concern. It dawns on me that his concern is probably less about me, or what I'm about to say, than about how it will affect him.

GO TO THE NEXT PAGE.

SoulCycle Scene, or What Happened Next:

Lights up on ME/JAMES (nonbinary, beautiful, twenty-seven), stands across from HIM (blond, rapist, somewhat older) in a SoulCycle. ME/JAMES's arms are crossed as if they are about to say something difficult (they are). HIM is leaning against the wall, listening intently.

*** Note from the playwright: For consistency, ME/JAMES should still be played by Cate Blanchett, Anne Hathaway, or Jessica Chastain. Casting HIM is a bit trickier. You need someone who is hot but also really loves sexual violence. Think Ted Bundy with a dye job or Ghislaine Maxwell before everything happened. If neither is available and you're a really fucked-up director (or just poor) you could have the same actor who played FINNEGAN play HIM, which would be both frightening and impactful.*

ME. So I have to be honest. We have met before, and I'd like to talk to you about that.

HIM. We have?

ME. Yeah. *(Beat.)* You don't remember?

HIM. Forgive me, I'm really trying—

ME. End of October, New York City . . .

HIM. Huh.

ME. You had just graduated from SoulCycle training.

HIM. Yeah, and then I moved here the next day . . .

ME. Exactly.

HIM. Did we meet that night?

ME. Yes. We did.

HIM. Oh, fuck, did we– *(He pauses, the sly grin returns.)* Did we fuck?

ME. That's not how I would say it.

HIM. Oh, shit, sorry.

ME. *(struck, because hearing the word "sorry" come out of HIM's mouth . . . means something)* We didn't hook up.

HIM. Gosh, I'm sorry, I'm really struggling to remem–

ME. You raped me.

HIM. I . . . . what?

ME. You raped me. That night.

(HIM looks at ME, unmoving.)

ME. I said no, but you didn't listen.

HIM. Wait a second here, that's a strong accu–

ME. It's not an accusation.

HIM. It's not?

ME. It's a fact.

HIM. Bro, listen, I'll be the first to admit I've done a lot of stuff with a lot of guys but I'm not a r—, a r— *(HIM can't say the word.)*

ME. A rapist?

HIM. Yeah, I'm not that.

ME. Unfortunately you are, and I have the medical records to prove it.

HIM. You what?

ME. I went to the doctor because I was bleeding. I had an internal anal fissure. It was so severe the doctors thought I might have to have surgery.

HIM. That's really awful, and I'm sorry that happened b—

ME. You're sorry that happened, or you're sorry you raped me?

HIM. Whoa now, I did NOT r-rape you. We agreed on doing—

ME. Oh, so now you remember.

HIM. Huh?

ME. We agreed on doing . . . ? That sounds like you just remembered something.

HIM. I mean, I remember that we hooked up, but I didn't . . . do that to you.

ME. So you lied.

HIM. What?

ME. When you said you didn't remember. You lied.

HIM. What? No! I didn't remember at first but now I remember you.

ME. So you remember raping me.

HIM. Jesus Christ, man!

ME. There's another thing; I'm not a man, actually.

HIM. What are you? Where did you come from? Why are you doing this?

"James?"

The scene is over. It was all in your head. You've been in your grandfather's kitchen the whole time. He's calling you.

GO TO PAGE 203.

I scurry around the corner of our ADA-compliant corridor that leads to my grandparents' bedroom. As a child I was rarely—if ever—allowed in here. Now, 6 years of Alzheimer's disease, 1 contractor, 1/2 a wall, and 439 wheelchair scuff marks on the floorboards later, I am a regular visitor.

My grandfather stares up at the ceiling where the fan trots rings above his head, like a faded halo. When my toes touch the carpet, I slow my pace so as not to startle him. The first waking moments are oft the most fragile; before reality can dust through the corners of his mind, dementia's residue will make his bedroom of nearly thirty years feel unfamiliar, make him want his mother, or render me a stranger.

His electric wheelchair is tucked next to his old reading chair across the room. Not that it needs to be so far away; he is nearly paralyzed from the waist down after a fall that wrung his spinal column like a wet towel. I try not to think about how his disability is a convenience for us, how it ensures his own safety. It feels cruel to note that if he were able to get himself out of bed and into his wheelchair unassisted it would pose a liability for everyone. At least when he is in bed I know he is safe, and he can't wander into danger (the yard, the street, who knows where else) with unsound mind. I pinch the chair's joystick and guide it toward the edge of his bed.

"Are you ready to get up, Grandpa?"

"Well, I sure am!" He smiles at the halo above. I feel grateful that whatever omnipotent being decided to poison his brain with dementia didn't have enough to reach the part that holds "childlike wonder" and "upbeat spirit."

I lift the covers and check his adult diaper (what a sentence). If he finds this undignified he never says so. I wonder if the omnipotent being in charge of killing our grandparents with this disease designed it to eliminate their shame around such matters, but I decide anything heinous enough to invent Alzheimer's lacked the compassion required to have this foresight. Luck of the draw. Fuck it all.

"Ok, I'm going to swing your legs over to the side of the bed so we can get you into your chair."

"Ok!"

"Here we go," I say, gripping his ankles firmly, and swing them over the side of the bed.

"Alright, I need you to pull on that bar and sit up." I point to the metal handle we attached to the bed years ago. It arcs like the railing on a community pool with the same silver sheen. His grip remains notably strong, and he hoists himself up to sitting.

"Perfect, now we're going to transfer into your chair."

"Alright!" He readies himself. I nudge the joystick and park perpendicular to the bed. We will now begin the most challenging part of the transfer: the ninety-degree pivot from bed to seat.

"You're gonna hold on to both of my hands." I kneel, sliding him into his house shoes and positioning his feet for the transfer. "And then twist toward me the whole time, and I'll tell you when to sit down."

He grips my hands with the same ferocity he offered the bar, and with great effort, he stands. For a second we are the same height, and he is my grandfather; sturdy, practiced, asking me what time we want to go to the bookstore and get a hot chocolate and a novel. Then his legs quiver and we are back in the delicacy of our pas de deux. The dance is tricky because he cannot bear much weight on his legs; he shuffles his feet until we have quarter-turned, and I cue him to sit. He lands in between the bars of the seat, grinning. Our hands separate. I exhale.

"Well," he says, adding the Appalachian-appropriate amount of syllables to the word. "Would you look at that!"

"Yes, that was great!" I bend down to secure his feet on his wheelchair's footrest.

"No, that!" He is pointing behind me. Outside the window one of the red birds, his favorite, hops along the windowsill.

He is laughing, and begins to twitter at the bird, who takes flight and soars out of view. My grandfather claps.

"Are you hungry?" I ask.

"You bet I am!"

"Is it . . ." He trails off, losing the word, and finally exclaims, "Breakfast!"

It is 5:17 p.m. There are vegetarian meatball subs and brussels sprouts waiting for him at the table.

"Yes, let's go get breakfast."

GO TO PAGE 205.

Everyone thinks it's a terrible idea, but I've decided to visit my rapist. I am afraid he doesn't know the severity of what he did to me. I'm afraid that he is raping other people and he doesn't know. I'm afraid he's doing well. I'm afraid I cannot hold the politic of restorative justice unless I practice it. I am afraid I am still attracted to him. I'm afraid of forgiving him. I'm afraid I can't forgive him. I'm afraid he will remember me. I'm afraid he won't. I'm afraid of him. I'm afraid of myself around him. I think the only way to overcome the fear is to go through it, and the only way I maintain a modicum of control is by visiting him in a public place. Somewhere it would be difficult to rape me. Again. I want our first interaction since the incident to be one I've prepared for. I don't want to be worried about running into him on the street. I don't want to keep running into his memory when other men touch me. I want control. I want to get this over with. I want to move on.

I rent a car. It's a 2022 Kia Soul. It looks like a toaster. I drive to his city. Hours later I pull into the parking lot. Neon signs flash SOULCYCLE. I put the car in park. Through the latticework windows is the famous studio emblem: a skull and crossbones.

I pull the key from the ignition. It snags on the windshield-wiper control. The windshield wipers begin frantically squeaking across the dash. It startles me. I turn them off. I place the keys in my pocket. I check myself out in the latticework windows. I pretend I like the reflection. Dread drains the life in my body. I tell myself I will not kill myself, no matter what he says or what happens. I will survive this. I will survive him. I am in control. I trust my body. I can do this.

I check in. He isn't there. I pick a bike. In the back. Lululemon moms. He comes in. He mounts the bike. He doesn't see me. ARE YOU READY TO SWEAT.

I am. He doesn't know it, but when I tell him why I'm here he'll be sweating too.

GO TO THE NEXT PAGE.

Scene at a Café Near a SoulCycle:

Lights up on ME/JAMES (nonbinary, beautiful, twenty-seven) in a café across from HIM (blond, rapist, somewhat older) near a SoulCycle. ME/JAMES sighs as if they are about to say something difficult (they are). HIM is sitting in his chair listening intently.

** *Note from the playwright: For consistency, ME/JAMES should still be played by Cate Blanchett, Anne Hathaway, or Jessica Chastain. Casting HIM is a bit trickier. In this moment it may be useful to employ men who look like remorseful golden retrievers, such as Jonathan Bailey or Shawn Mendes, if he can act. If neither is available and you're a really fucked-up director (or just poor) you could have the same actor who played FINNEGAN play HIM, which would be both frightening and impactful.*

ME. Thanks for meeting me here.

HIM. Yeah of course.

(A long pause.)

HIM. So . . .

ME. So I don't know if you remember when we met . . .

HIM. I actually do, it was the night before I moved here, right?

ME. Yeah, it was.

HIM. I mean, it's good to see you, I guess, I'm just a little confused as to—

ME. *(blurting it out)* You raped me.

HIM. I . . . . what?

ME. Yeah. I'm sorry, I didn't know how to tell you.

HIM. Oh my god.

ME. Yeah.

HIM. There's no way.

ME. Well, actually–

HIM. I mean–

ME. See I knew I shoul–

HIM. Did I really?

(HIM looks genuinely concerned. ME/JAMES softens.)

ME. Yeah, you really did.

(Another pause. They both shift uncomfortably.)

HIM. James, I am genuinely so sorry.

ME. What?

HIM. I am so, so, sorry. That must have been awful.

ME. You believe me?

HIM. To be honest I'm still processing. That's a really strong thing to say but I can't imagine you drove all the way here over nothing. If you say I did that then something must've happened.

ME. Do you remember what happened?

HIM. I . . . really don't.

ME. Well, I asked you to stop and . . .

HIM. And I didn't, did I?

ME. *(Shakes their head. Being believed is hard.)* No, you didn't. I'm sorry for bringing this up—

HIM. I don't think this will make it any better, but I was in a really difficult place in my life then. I wasn't respecting myself, and I definitely wasn't respecting other people. I wish I could remember what happened, but I don't, and that means you're probably right. Fuck. Fuck.

ME.

HIM.

ME.

HIM.

ME.

HIM. Are you . . . are you gonna press charges?

ME. No, no, that's not what this is about.

HIM. Christ, sorry, I shouldn't be thinking about me in this moment. See, there I go again! Always thinking of myself. I should've asked if you were ok or how you possibly managed these last years or like . . . how did you . . .

ME. I'm ok.

HIM. You are?

ME. Well, it was really bad for a while. I could tell something was going on at the time because your eyes lost all their color when you finished.

HIM. My therapist says that's what happens when I dissociate.

ME. You're in therapy?

HIM. Yeah. I started a few years back. I'm trying to own my mistakes.

ME. That's really big of you.

HIM. I hurt a guy a while back. My ex. Well, my boyfriend then. He actually told me a kind of similar story from when we were together. I don't know why I'm telling you this—

ME. So there were others?

HIM. I guess so. One other, at least.

ME. How is he?

HIM. *(without eye contact)* I don't really know. I think he's ok. He blocked me, after everything. I hurt him badly and I regret it every day. We don't talk anymore and I wish I could make things better but I just, I can't.

(HIM is crying. ME/JAMES unfreezes and pulls a napkin from the dispenser at the table. They offer it to HIM.)

HIM. Thank you.

(ME/JAMES nods.)

HIM. No, I mean thank you for telling me. I am so deeply sorry for what I did to you, and to him. My therapist told me that becoming a better person would mean facing the reality of who I used to be and I guess this is who I used to be.

ME.

HIM. I know I can't fix the past. And I know I can't fix things with him. Or you. Because what I did was unforgivable. I wish I could go back in time and slap me in the face and say, "That's a human being, you know! A real, live human being and they deserve respect." But my therapist also says we can't control the past, only our reactions in the present.

ME. You have a good therapist.

HIM. And I promise you that I will do everything I can to act in accordance to my values in the future. I'll never do what I did to you to anyone else ever again.

(HIM is barely holding it together. ME/JAMES is still, taking it in. This is all they've wanted to hear for the past five years. An apology, an admission of guilt, accountability, a plan for change. Hearing the words out loud they seem so small. So quiet. HIM seems so small.)

HIM. I'm in a support group, actually.

ME. You are?

HIM. Yeah, with other guys who have . . . similar stories. We call ourselves the Upstanders. It's kinda corny but we are trying to live the values of being upstanding citizens and telling other guys about this so they don't, you know, repeat the cycle.

ME. You're doing that?

HIM. Yeah, I am. They're really good guys, actually. I know that might not be right to say to you, but they are.

ME. I . . . I don't really know what to say. That's amazing. I didn't know those groups existed.

HIM. Yeah, I didn't either. More guys need to know about them, I guess. I wish I'd found it before I met you.

ME. Yeah, me too.

(Another pause. Neither is sure what to say.)

HIM. I know sorry doesn't change anything. But I am sorry. And I promise you, I promise you I'll never do something like that again.

ME. *(a glimmer)* I hope you're right.

(ME/JAMES begins gathering their things. She stands, looks at HIM, and briefly considers what to do next. The actress playing ME/JAMES should follow their instincts—does she offer another napkin? A hug? A

few parting words? What feels right in this moment? Does anything? Once she makes the choice ME/JAMES exits. HIM remains on stage in the silence.)

"James?"

The scene is over. It was all in your head. You've been in your grandfather's kitchen the whole time. He's calling you.

GO TO PAGE 193.

Everyone thinks it's a terrible idea, but I've decided to visit my rapist. I am afraid he doesn't know the severity of what he did to me. I'm afraid that he is raping other people and he doesn't know. I'm afraid he's doing well. I'm afraid I cannot hold the politic of restorative justice unless I practice it. I am afraid I am still attracted to him. I'm afraid of forgiving him. I'm afraid I can't forgive him. I'm afraid he will remember me. I'm afraid he won't. I'm afraid of him. I'm afraid of myself around him. I think the only way to overcome the fear is to go through it, and the only way I maintain a modicum of control is by visiting him in a public place. Somewhere it would be difficult to rape me. Again. I want our first interaction since the incident to be one I've prepared for. I don't want to be worried about running into him on the street. I don't want to keep running into his memory when other men touch me. I want control. I want to get this over with. I want to move on.

I rent a car. It's a 2022 Kia Soul. It looks like a toaster. I drive to his city. Hours later I pull into the parking lot. Neon signs flash SOUL-CYCLE. I put the car in park. Through the latticework windows is the famous studio emblem: a skull and crossbones.

I pull the key from the ignition. It snags on the windshield-wiper control. The windshield wipers begin frantically squeaking across the dash. It startles me. I turn them off. I place the keys in my pocket. I check myself out in the latticework windows. I pretend I like the reflection. Dread drains the life in my body. I tell myself I will not kill myself, no matter what he says or what happens. I will survive this. I will survive him. I am in control. I trust my body. I can do this.

I enter the lobby of the studio. He isn't there. I check in. I choose a bike in the back between a Lululemon-wrapped soccer mom and a college sophomore on his first week of Accutane. A ponytail with purple leggings sits in the first row, directly in front of the instructor bike. I hate her because she feels comfortable being so close to him.

"Heeeyyy, welcome!" The door swings open. It's him: black shirt, black shorts, headset balanced in his ears. The left ear is one-eighth of an inch higher than the right. He adjusts the headset and smiles at Ponytail. They hug. I hate her because he's nice to her. His biceps bubble at the elbow, just enough to say, "I lift less than I cycle," but "One time I held down this hot nonbinary girl and didn't listen to her when she said no." Ponytail says something. His eyes crinkle, he laughs, he closes the studio door.

I'm taller than he is. I had forgotten this, or I didn't know, because we didn't spend much time standing. He's the kind of blond where his eyelashes are thick and invisible at the same time. His left incisor is capped with tiny ridges that look like the letter *m* on repeat. I'm meeting my other half, again. The other half of every therapy session, every nightmare, every tear-stricken moment of attempted intimacy with a man for the last five years. He's gorgeous. I wonder if he really is the same person.

He mounts the instructor bike in the center of the studio like a swordsman mounting a horse before battle. He serenades the room of Lululemon-wrapped soccer moms, sophomores on Accutane, and Ponytails with a cheesy, "take it at your own pace" speech buttoned with "ARE YOU READY TO SWEAT?"

I am. He doesn't know it, but if I told him why I'm here he'd be sweating too.

The music starts. He leans forward on his bike. His hands grip the foam-coated handlebars. Suddenly it is October, I am underneath him, and his handlebars are my shoulders. The music dampens, his breathing quickens, and I feel sweat on my brow. His incisor gleams. The candles flicker. I hear screaming. Then I'm back in the studio, and I realize the screaming is coming from Lululemon to my left because I've just vomited on her bike.

"James?"

The scene is over. It was all in your head. You've been in your grandfather's kitchen the whole time. He's calling you.

GO TO PAGE 201.

I scurry around the corner of our ADA-compliant corridor that leads to my grandparents' bedroom. As a child I was rarely—if ever—allowed in here. Now, 6 years of Alzheimer's disease, 1 contractor, 1/2 a wall, and 438 wheelchair scuff marks on the floorboards later, I am a regular visitor.

My grandfather stares up at the ceiling where the fan trots rings above his head, like a faded halo. When my toes touch the carpet, I slow my pace so as not to startle him. The first waking moments are oft the most fragile; before reality can dust through the corners of his mind, dementia's residue will make his bedroom of nearly thirty years feel unfamiliar, make him want his mother, or render me a stranger.

His electric wheelchair is tucked next to his old reading chair across the room. Not that it needs to be so far away; he is nearly paralyzed from the waist down after a fall that wrung his spinal column like a wet towel. I try not to think about how his disability is a convenience for us, how it ensures his own safety. It feels cruel to note that if he were able to get himself out of bed and into his wheelchair unassisted it would pose a liability for everyone. When he is in bed I know he is safe, and he can't wander into danger (the yard, the street, who knows where else) with unsound mind. I pinch the chair's joystick and guide it toward the edge of his bed.

"Are you ready to get up, Grandpa?"

"Well, I sure am!" He smiles at the halo above. I feel grateful that whatever omnipotent being decided to poison his brain with dementia didn't have enough to reach the part that holds "childlike wonder" and "upbeat spirit."

I lift the covers and check his adult diaper (what a sentence). If he finds this undignified he never says so. I wonder if the omnipotent being in charge of killing our grandparents with this disease designed it to eliminate their shame around such matters, but I decide anything heinous enough to invent Alzheimer's lacked the compassion required to have this foresight. Luck of the draw. Fuck it all.

"Ok, I'm going to swing your legs over to the side of the bed so we can get you into your chair."

"Sure." Today he seems to know the routine.

"Here we go," I say, gripping his ankles firmly and swinging them over the side of the bed.

"Alright, I need you to pull on that bar and sit up." I point to the metal handle we attached to the bed years ago. It arcs like the railing on a community pool with the same silver sheen. His grip remains notably strong, and he hoists himself up to sitting.

"Perfect, now we're going to transfer into your chair."

"Alright!" He nods. I nudge the joystick and park perpendicular to the bed. We will now begin the most challenging part of the transfer: the ninety-degree pivot from bed to seat.

"You're gonna hold on to both of my hands." I kneel, sliding him into his house shoes and positioning his feet for the transfer. "And then twist toward me the whole time, and I'll tell you when to sit down."

He grips my hands with the same ferocity he offered the bar, and with great effort, he stands. Then he falters, and lands back down on the bed.

"It's ok," I say. "We'll try again when you're ready."

He offers me his hands again, and this time he stands. For a second we are the same height, and he is my grandfather; sturdy, practiced, asking me what time we want to go to the bookstore and get a hot chocolate and a novel. Then his legs quiver and we are back in the delicacy of our pas de deux. The dance is tricky because he cannot bear much weight on his legs; he shuffles his feet until we have quarter-turned, and I spot a rogue shoelace threatening his left foot, the one he is about to shuffle. Dammit. If he falls, I am not strong enough to pick him back up. If he sits now, he may hit his hip on the armchair. I cut my losses early and without looking at the chair I cue him to sit. His hip bone collides with the armchair, knocking him onto the seat cushion. He inhales, sharply.

"Well," he says, adding the Appalachian-appropriate amount of syllables to the word.

"I'm sorry you hit your hip, that was my fault."

He dismisses my apology with the wave of his hand. "You are a very helpful young man!"

I smile, and not out of habit, but because he has always called me this. I will accept being a young man to my grandfather in this moment alone because the wheelchair transfer was hard today and he has a degenerative brain condition and when he calls me a young man it means he recognizes me and I have not been lost to the bowels of dementia, not yet. I flip my hair behind my shoulders and bend down to retie his shoelace.

"Thank you," I say as his grandson. "Are you hungry, Grandpa?"

"I certainly am!"

It is 5:16 p.m. There is broccoli rabe with penne, mustard sauce, and deviled eggs waiting for him at the table.

"Let's go eat."

GO TO THE NEXT PAGE.

Everyone thinks it's a terrible idea, but I've decided to visit my rapist. I am afraid he doesn't know the severity of what he did to me. I'm afraid that he is raping other people and he doesn't know. I'm afraid he's doing well. I'm afraid I cannot hold the politic of restorative justice unless I practice it. I am afraid I am still attracted to him. I'm afraid of forgiving him. I'm afraid I can't forgive him. I'm afraid he will remember me. I'm afraid he won't. I'm afraid of him. I'm afraid of myself around him. I think the only way to overcome the fear is to go through it, and the only way I maintain a modicum of control is by visiting him in a public place. Somewhere it would be difficult to rape me. Again. I want our first interaction since the incident to be one I've prepared for. I don't want to be worried about running into him on the street. I don't want to keep running into his memory when other men touch me. I want control. I want to get this over with. I want to move on.

I rent a car. It's a 2022 Kia Soul. It looks like a toaster. I drive to his city. Hours later I pull into the parking lot. Neon signs flash SOUL-CYCLE. I put the car in park. Through the latticework windows is the famous studio emblem: a skull and crossbones.

I pull the key from the ignition. It snags on the windshield-wiper control. The windshield wipers begin frantically squeaking across the dash. It startles me. I turn them off. I place the keys in my pocket. I check myself out in the latticework windows. I pretend I like the reflection. Dread drains the life in my body. I tell myself I will not kill myself, no matter what he says or what happens. I will survive this. I will survive him. I am in control. I trust my body. I can do this.

I check in. He isn't there. I pick a bike. In the back. Lululemon moms. He comes in. He mounts the bike. He doesn't see me. ARE YOU READY TO SWEAT.

***

I was, in fact, ready and I did, in fact, sweat through my entire ensemble while riding an overpriced stationary bike for fifty-five minutes accompanied by the backbeat of Taylor Swift's "Anti-Hero" (the version featuring Bleachers, which I do honestly think is the superior remix, with the ILLENIUM a close second) and the motivational voice of my rapist. I have brought a change of clothes and I dash into the locker room. I choose the men's, mostly because I'm afraid one of the Lululemon moms is a TERF. The locker room is empty. I exhale.

I've made it this far. I saw him, and I did not die. I did not want to kill myself. I laughed, even! His corny lines of encouragement, the headset mic cutting out mid Kim Petras chorus, the fact that his highest pedestal is a bike that goes nowhere. I grab a towel and lay my change of clothes on the farthest bench from the door. I check my phone: I have enough time to shower off and drive home before it's dark. I peel my sticky clothes and discard them into a plastic bag, wrapping the towel around my waist. I'm almost done.

"Hey, cutie."

I turn. Black shoes, black shorts, left incisor, tiny *m*'s.

"Sorry," he puts his hands out. "I didn't mean to startle you!" He is eight lockers away from my bench. He fingers the lock in front of him. Fingers that once felt like screws. It springs open. He pulls his shirt clean over his head and hangs it on the locker door.

"Are you just gonna stare?" He grins, the incisor melts to the width of his smile. Like an orange slice. His chest hair blooms from his sternum. I must have been staring.

"Oh, sorry, I just—" I'm white-knuckling my towel. I feel topless, as if I should've wrapped the towel around my chest so he couldn't see the favors estrogen has been doing me. He is also topless but for him it's shirtless, I guess? His thumbs threaten the waistband of the black shorts.

He hooks them under the elastic. "You just what?"

I look away.

"No, it's ok, you can look. But be careful, look too long and you'll see me naked!"

I blush. I have seen him naked. I've seen men that look like him naked. I've seen hundreds, even thousands of men naked. I don't know why I'm blushing.

"Sorry, I guess I should introduce myself." He extends a hand. "You know, start this properly."

Properly. I don't know what to do so I shake it. We exchange names. He uses a nickname, a shortened version from last time, the first time, when he shortened the lifecycle of my nervous system.

"You were in class, weren't you?"

"Yeah, um, I was."

"You did really well." He folds the black shirt and stuffs it in a plastic bag.

"Oh, thanks. You're a good teacher. Instructor? I don't know what to call it. You. You're not an *it,* you're a you, and that's what I mean." I am floundering.

"You can call me whatever you want." He pauses. "As long as you call me."

I roll my eyes with a reflexive "Oh, Christ." I can feel my cheeks redden.

"What, I'm not allowed to want you to call me?"

You already have my number, I want to say, but I am distracted by his thumbs teasing his waistband again.

"I hope I'm not making you uncomfortable. You're just really cute."

"Oh, er—thanks." I almost smile. This is all so unexpected. He is supposed to be a rapist, not a cheesy flirt.

Without breaking eye contact he sends the black shorts down his legs, kicks them into his palm with one hand, and adjusts his briefs with the other. They're deep purple, puckering in all the right places around the package underneath. He flexes, and the muscles of his stomach knot into ropy squares. He shifts his weight to one leg, quadricep bulging as he discards the shorts into the plastic bag.

"Enjoying the view?"

"W-what?"

"Because you're hard as a rock."

I break our gaze to look down. To my horror I have pitched a tent in my towel, but much to the amusement of the man dangerously close to shedding his purple briefs in front of me. I turn around and scramble to tuck my dick into the folds of the fabric.

"Hey, it's ok, it's normal. I mean, I'm getting hard looking at you too."

I pause. He continues. The purple pucker twitches.

"Listen, you can look away anytime if you don't want to see . . ."

Tent intact, I want to watch him pull his purple briefs down and step out of them. He stares at me. I like his staring. I decide to return the favor and let the towel slip from my fingers. It joins his briefs on my side of the floor.

"Oops," I whisper.

"Holy fuck," he says. He's already fondling himself. His knees slacken as he strokes.

He wants me. He's attracted to me, he's aroused because of me, he can't take his eyes off me. It is so different this time.

"You like what you see?" I take a step toward him. I have the chance to fix everything.

"Oh yeah, baby." His voice is quiet now. A whisper.

"You want this?" Another step, then another. My tip is inches from his. He reaches out a hand and cups my waist. His touch feels like fireworks. He slides it behind and grabs my ass.

"I want this," he breathes.

And then I'm kissing him. He is up against the locker, both hands on my butt, his cock tucked in between my own and my inner thigh. My tongue pushes past the incisor and he tastes like freedom.

"You're so fucking sexy," he pants.

"Thanks, you are too." And I mean it, he is. His hand has made its way up my spine to cradle the back of my neck. It feels nice to be held this way: firm, tender, attentive. Maybe he wasn't always what I thought he was. Maybe I am remembering it all incorrectly. Maybe he was always gentle and I just didn't know how to accept that gentleness because I wanted it to go a certain way and it didn't and I couldn't pivot and if I'd have just pivoted maybe I would've enjoyed it because he is hot and he does want me and if I'd just relaxed a little like Kyren I could've avoided all this. Maybe it was always good and I just got confused.

"Do you want to?" He bites at my neck. I moan. "Because we don't have to if you don't want t—"

"I want to." I breathe. I want him and I want it to feel good.

He pulls me into the showers. The water is hot and I can't wait to have the taste of freedom on my tongue again. He presses me up against the tile wall and bites at my lip. My fingers and the water meet at his hairline. He pumps conditioner into his hand and rubs it between my legs.

"Are you ready?"

I turn around. Shower-doggy. I arch my back. He kisses my shoulder. I'm ready. I'm ready to feel connected to him, ready to feel his undivided attention, ready for him to tell me how good I feel. I'm ready for him to hold my backside into his chest and ask if I want it faster or slower and kiss me while he cums. I'm ready and I want it and when he does it—all of it—I feel the pain evaporate from my body.

"You're so fucking beautiful," he whispers, and he means it. "Where have you been all my life?"

This is it. This is who he really is. This is what I always wanted. It is possible to erase bad experiences if you mark them with new ones. Better ones. Like this one. This is how it was supposed to feel the first time.

And then, as it always happens, I start to cry. He pulls out with a conditioner-soaked squelch and I'm mortified and I hide my face in my hands. He turns the water off. My vision crackles. I teeter. He catches me by the shoulders as I slump to the floor. If he says anything I don't hear it. Catharsis overtakes. I am a ball against the shower wall. Water, slimed with conditioner, slithers through my leg hair and drains with a gurgle and a belch. When I can breathe again I open my eyes, knowing he will be gone. Instead, there he is, hunched over, hands cupping my face, his eyes the color of a glacier as it rolls back into the arctic sea. I look away. He takes me by the chin, thumbing me back to center so I face him.

"I just knew you were gonna cry." He grins. "I just knew it."

"James?"

The scene is over. It was all in your head. You've been in your grandfather's kitchen the whole time. He's calling you.

GO TO PAGE 181.

I scurry around the corner of our ADA-compliant corridor that leads to my grandparents' bedroom. As a child I was rarely—if ever—allowed in here. Now, 6 years of Alzheimer's disease, 1 contractor, 1/2 a wall, and 437 wheelchair scuff marks on the floorboards later, I am a regular visitor.

My grandfather stares up at the ceiling where the fan trots rings above his head, like a faded halo. When my toes touch the carpet, I slow my pace so as not to startle him. The first waking moments are oft the most fragile; before reality can dust through the corners of his mind, dementia's residue will make his bedroom of nearly thirty years feel unfamiliar, make him want his mother, or render me a stranger.

His electric wheelchair is tucked next to his old reading chair across the room. Not that it needs to be so far away; he is nearly paralyzed from the waist down after a fall that wrung his spinal column like a wet towel. I try not to think about how his disability is a convenience for us, how it ensures his own safety. It feels cruel to note that if he were able to get himself out of bed and into his wheelchair unassisted it would pose a liability for everyone. When he is in bed I know he is safe, and he can't wander into danger (the yard, the street, who knows where else) with unsound mind. I pinch the chair's joystick and guide it toward the edge of his bed.

"Are you ready to get up, Grandpa?"

"Well, I sure am!" He smiles at the halo above. I feel grateful that whatever omnipotent being decided to poison his brain with dementia didn't have enough to reach the part that holds "childlike wonder" and "upbeat spirit."

I lift the covers and check his adult diaper (what a sentence). If he finds this undignified he never says so. I wonder if the omnipotent being in charge of killing our grandparents with this disease designed it to eliminate their shame around such matters, but I decide anything heinous enough to invent Alzheimer's lacked the compassion required to have this foresight. Luck of the draw. Fuck it all.

"Ok, I'm going to swing your legs over to the side of the bed so we can get you into your chair."

"Well, if you say so!" Today the routine is a surprise.

"Yes," I say, gripping his ankles firmly and swinging them over the side of the bed.

"Alright, I need you to pull on that bar and sit up." I point to the metal handle we attached to the bed years ago. It arcs like the railing on a community pool with the same silver sheen. His grip remains notably strong, and he hoists himself up to sitting.

"Perfect, now we're going to transfer into your chair."

"Are you sure about that?" He chuckles.

"Yes, we did it earlier today! I promise it works." I nudge the joystick and park perpendicular to the bed. We will now begin the most challenging part of the transfer: the ninety-degree pivot from bed to seat.

"You're gonna hold on to both of my hands." I kneel, sliding him into his house shoes and positioning his feet for the transfer. "And then twist toward me the whole time, and I'll tell you when to sit down."

He grips my hands with the same ferocity he offered the bar, and with great effort, he stands. For a second we are the same height, and he is my grandfather; sturdy, practiced, asking me what time we want to go to the bookstore and get a hot chocolate and a novel. Then his legs quiver and we are back in the delicacy of our pas de deux. The dance is tricky because he cannot bear much weight on his legs; he shuffles his feet until we have quarter-turned, and his foot gets stuck.

"Can you lift your foot? I think it might be stuck."

He winces and manages to shift enough weight to right his foot.

"There you go." I peer over our joint elbows to double-check: If I guide his fall he will land squarely between the armrests of his wheelchair.

"Alright, you can sit down." I use the momentum of his drop to angle him over just enough so both hips clear the bar. He plops onto his seat, grinning. Our hands separate. I exhale.

"Well," he says, adding the Appalachian-appropriate amount of syllables to the word. "That's that!"

His face scrunches and I know he's about to ask a question.

"Is it time for . . . ?"

"For dinner?"

"Dinner! Yes!"

It is 5:15 p.m. There is broccoli cheddar soup and homemade bread waiting for him at the table.

"Yes, let's go get dinner."

GO TO PAGE 183.

I scurry around the corner of our ADA-compliant corridor that leads to my grandparents' bedroom. As a child I was rarely—if ever—allowed in here. Now, 6 years of Alzheimer's disease, 1 contractor, 1/2 a wall, and 436 wheelchair scuff marks on the floorboards later, I am a regular visitor.

My grandfather stares up at the ceiling where the fan trots rings above his head, like a faded halo. When my toes touch the carpet, I slow my pace so as not to startle him. The first waking moments are oft the most fragile; before reality can dust through the corners of his mind, dementia's residue will make his bedroom of nearly thirty years feel unfamiliar, make him want his mother, or render me a stranger.

His electric wheelchair is tucked next to his old reading chair across the room. Not that it needs to be so far away; he is nearly paralyzed from the waist down after a fall that wrung his spinal column like a wet towel. I try not to think about how his disability is a convenience for us, how it ensures his own safety. It feels cruel to note that if he were able to get himself out of bed and into his wheelchair unassisted it would pose a liability for everyone. When he is in bed I know he is safe, and he can't wander into danger (the yard, the street, who knows where else) with unsound mind. I pinch the chair's joystick and guide it toward the edge of his bed.

"Are you ready to get up, Grandpa?"

"Well, I sure am!" He smiles at the halo above. I feel grateful that whatever omnipotent being decided to poison his brain with dementia didn't have enough to reach the part that holds "childlike wonder" and "upbeat spirit."

I lift the covers and check his adult diaper (what a sentence). If he finds this undignified he never says so. I wonder if the omnipotent being in charge of killing our grandparents with this disease designed it to eliminate their shame around such matters, but I decide anything heinous enough to invent Alzheimer's lacked the compassion required to have this foresight. Luck of the draw. Fuck it all.

"Ok, I'm going to swing your legs over to the side of the bed so we can get you into your chair."

"Really now!" Today the routine is as much of a surprise to him as his burst of energy is to me.

"Yes," I say, gripping his ankles firmly and swinging them over the side of the bed.

"Alright, I need you to pull on that bar and sit up." I point to the metal handle we attached to the bed years ago. It arcs like the railing on a community pool with the same silver sheen. His grip remains notably strong, and he hoists himself up to sitting.

"Perfect, now we're going to transfer into your chair."

"Alright!" he claps. I nudge the joystick and park perpendicular to the bed. We will now begin the most challenging part of the transfer: the ninety-degree pivot from bed to seat.

"You're gonna hold on to both of my hands." I kneel, sliding him into his house shoes and positioning his feet for the transfer. "And then twist toward me the whole time, and I'll tell you when to sit down."

He grips my hands with the same ferocity he offered the bar, and with great effort, he stands. For a second we are the same height, and he is my grandfather; sturdy, practiced, asking me what time we want to go to the bookstore and get a hot chocolate and a novel. Then his legs quiver and we are back in the delicacy of our pas de deux. The dance is tricky because he cannot bear much weight on his legs; he shuffles his feet until we have quarter-turned, and I cue him to sit. He lands in between the bars of the seat, grinning. Our hands separate. I exhale.

"Well," he says, adding the Appalachian-appropriate amount of syllables to the word. "Let's go get breakfast!"

It is 5:14 p.m. There are veggie burgers and roasted asparagus waiting for him at the table.

"Yes, let's go get breakfast."

GO TO PAGE 191.

Everyone thinks it's a terrible idea, but I've decided to visit my rapist. Afraid he doesn't know the severity. Afraid that he is raping other people. Afraid he's doing well. Afraid I cannot hold the politic of restorative justice unless I practice it. Afraid I am still attracted to him. Afraid of forgiving him. Afraid I can't forgive him. Afraid he will remember me. Afraid he won't. Afraid of him. Afraid of myself around him. Only way to overcome the fear is to go through it. Only modicum of control is by visiting him in public. Somewhere it would be difficult to rape me. Again. I want our first interaction since the incident to be one I've prepared for. Don't want to be worried about running into him on the street. Don't want to keep running into his memory when other men touch me. Control. Get this over with. Move on.

Rent car. Kia Soul. Toaster. Drive. Parking lot. SOULCYCLE. Park. Skull and crossbones.

Pull the key. Windshield wipers. Turn them off. Keys in my pocket. Pretend I like the reflection. Dread drains the life in my body. I tell myself I will not kill myself, no matter what he says or what happens. Survive this. Survive him. Control. Trust my body. Do this.

I check in. He isn't there. I pick a bike. In the back. Lululemon moms. He comes in. He mounts the bike. He doesn't see me. ARE YOU READY TO SWEAT.

***

I was ready and I did sweat. I have brought a change of clothes and I dash into the locker room. I choose the men's. (TERFs.) The locker room is empty.

I've made it this far. I grab a towel and lay my change of clothes out. I check my phone. Enough time to shower off and drive home before it's dark. I'm almost done.

"Hey, cutie."

I turn. Black shoes, black shorts, left incisor, tiny *m*'s.

"Sorry, I didn't mean to startle you!" He pulls his shirt clean over his head. "Are you just gonna stare?" I must have been staring.

"Oh, sorry, I just—" I'm white-knuckling my towel.

His thumbs threaten the waistband of the black shorts. I look away.

"It's ok, you can look."

I blush. I don't know why I'm blushing.

"But be careful, look too long and you'll see me naked!"

Without breaking eye contact he sends the black shorts down his legs, kicks them into his palm with one hand, and adjusts his briefs with the other. They're deep purple, puckering in all the right places around the package underneath. He flexes, and the muscles of his stomach knot into ropy squares. The ropy squares bend, and the purple briefs land in a heap on the floor. He discards both items into the plastic bag. He stands in front of me, buck naked.

"You know, now that you've seen me, I should probably see you naked too. Fair is fair."

He paws at his junk and waits, as if he expects me to drop my towel. When I don't he shrugs and shoulders past me to the showers. I hear the shower water.

Fair is fair.

I have an idea. I turn toward the showers, and he watches me take the stall directly across from him. I make a show of sliding the towel off my backside and bending over to start the water. I step in and begin to smooth the water down my body from my shoulders down to my ankles.

I turn around and he's stroking.

"Fuck yeah," he mouths.

"Yeah?" I say with an eyebrow raise.

His knees slacken as he grips himself. His lips part. He wants me. This is what I want. I remember that look, the greed, the narrowed eyes, the all-consuming devotion to his own pleasure. Only this time I'm not pinned underneath him, I'm in a shower stall across from him, tantalizing him with my body. *Fair is fair.* I beckon him into my stall.

"I knew you'd come around," he says, closing the glass door behind him.

"Oh, did you?"

"Yeah," he leans in, snaking his hands around my back. One clutches my ass, then smacks it. "Besides, you're lucky. Not everyone gets to play with me."

"Oh, I'm lucky, am I?"

"Oh, yeah." The other cheek, another smack. "I'm gonna change your life."

I can't help it, I laugh.

"What's so funny?"

"Oh, nothing." I wrap my arms around him, preparing for a kiss. He's in perfect position. "It's just . . . you already have."

Right as our lips are about to meet I grab a fistful of hair and smash his head into the tile wall. It cracks, or his forehead does. I pull him back up. Blood spills from his nostrils like it spilled out of me and into my bathtub five years ago. I grip his hair harder and slam his face against the wall again. Blood sprays across the tile on contact and by the third time I hear him scream. He is clawing at me, but I'm wet and he can't get a good grip. I yank his head back to inspect my work. His lip is split down to his chin, his eyes are rolling back. Blood pools in his mouth. He gags, and I jackknife his head forward so the blood plops onto the thick rubber mat. He manages one good punch against my rib cage. I double back, hit the shower wall, and almost lose my grip on his hair. I knee him in the groin, reducing him to all fours. Another scream. He's going to attract attention. While he's doubled over I grab the conditioner bottle and bludgeon it into his mouth. It muffles the next scream, but not enough. It slips out on a landslide of blood, and something shiny clatters onto the drain grate. The incisor.

"You know why I'm here, and you know what you did," I bark.

"Whatdidi—whatdidi—" he chokes, spits, whimpers.

"You don't remember?"

He cowers in the fetal position, limbs knocking against the tile wall, looking at me as if he truly doesn't.

I tower over him. He winces. "Five years ago you raped me."

His eyes widen, and I know he remembers. He spits again. Another tooth. He might be crying or panting, I can't tell. I don't care. He didn't. Fair is fair.

"Well if I did," he wheezes. "Then you fucking deserved it."

Then I fucking deserved it.

He makes a move as if he's going to attempt standing. I curb stomp his jaw. He screams again, and when I remove my heel there's a dent in the crimson-stained stubble where it has dislocated. He starts to cry. Heavy, pathetic, siren-like wails. I know it's only a matter of time before someone hears.

I think about every time I've lain in that exact same position, crying myself to sleep because I too was bleeding. I think about how many other people he forced himself onto and into and how he probably told them they were "lucky" or they "deserved" it. I think about how many moments of joy and solitude and peace he's stolen from me and who knows how many other people and all I feel is rage redder than the pool of liquid under his cheek. I think about how rape is never justifiable but murder sometimes is. And I think of how much better and safer the world would be with one less predator, and before I know it I have the conditioner bottle in my hand and stabbed him in the neck with the nozzle.

The first stab doesn't puncture, but his wailing intensifies. I think of how I wailed and he refused to stop, so I return the favor. I line the metal point with his neck and punch it from above like a sledgehammer. It penetrates, an action he is all too familiar with. It squirts like a geyser. For some reason I know to pull down, tearing the skin from where his jaw used to be down to his clavicle. I ignore his screaming and the gushing down the drain from his neck's spillage and I hack away at the arteries, veins, the ability to rape people, until he stops.

Then he is still. I don't have to check, I know it's over. It's silent. The drain is clogged by teeth and flesh chunks and other unidentifiable matter that kept him alive long enough to ruin people's lives. With his neck split like a pig at the butcher shop on the floor of a SoulCycle shower he doesn't seem so powerful anymore. I chuckle. He looks like a frog after a botched high school dissection. I am sure I look horrible. I reach up to smooth my hair, but feel something squish. I wash my hand under the shower, which is still running. Scarlet water flecked with tissue slithers through my leg hair and drains with a gurgle and a belch. It's over. I did it. I am probably supposed to feel remorse for murdering someone but all I feel is relief. I did what I had to. I protected my community. I protected myself. Fair is now fair. Murder can be justifiable. Rape cannot. I stopped it from getting worse. I am a hero. I am—

"James?"

The scene is over. It was all in your head. You've been in your grandfather's kitchen the whole time. He's calling you.

GO TO PAGE 211.

Scurry around the corner, 446 scuff marks, regular visitor

Ceiling, faded halo, wheelchair joystick, "Are you ready to get up, Grandpa?"

Check diaper

(What a sentence)

Swing his legs over the side of the bed

Grab handle

Community pool

Chair transfer: ninety-degree pivot

"Hold both of my hands"

ShuffleshuffleshuffleshufflepausecheckshuffleSIT

5:23

"Let's go get breakfast"

GO TO PAGE 215.

Everyone thinks it's a terrible idea, but I've decided to visit my rapist.

Severity / raping other people / doing well / cannot hold the politic of restorative justice unless I practice it. Still attracted to him? Forgive him? Can't forgive him? Will remember me, won't remember me, afraid of him, myself around him, only way out is through. In public. Control. Get this over with. Move on.

Rent car. Kia Soul. Toaster. Drive. Parking lot. SOULCYCLE. Park. Skull and crossbones.

Pull the key. Windshield wipers. Turn them off. Keys in my pocket. Pretend I like the reflection. Dread drains the life in my body. I tell myself I will not kill myself, no matter what he says or what happens. Survive this. Survive him. Control. Trust my body. Do this.

"James?"

The scene is over.

GO TO PAGE 213.

He didn't call you.

GO TO PAGE 210.

I check in. He isn't there. I pick a bike. In the back. Lululemon moms. Someone else comes in. I don't recognize them. They are not my rapist. They mount the bike. They are subbing for my rapist who is stuck in traffic. I am equal parts disappointed and relieved. ARE YOU READY TO SWEAT.

"James?"

GO TO PAGE 209.

I scurry around the corner of our ADA-compliant corridor, rarely allowed, 442 scuff marks, regular visitor.

My grandfather stares up at the ceiling, fan trots rings, faded halo, first waking moments are the most fragile.

His electric wheelchair is tucked next to his old reading chair, so far away, disability, pinch the chair's joystick, "Are you ready to get up, Grandpa?"

Childlike wonder, upbeat spirit.

Check diaper. (What a sentence)

"Ok, I'm going to swing your legs over to the side of the bed so we can get you into your chair."

Grip his ankles firmly and swing them over the side of the bed.

"Alright, I need you to pull on that bar and sit up."

Hoists himself up to sitting. Community pool,

Chair transfer:

"Hold both of my hands."

For a second we are the same height, and he is my grandfather; sturdy, practiced, asking me what time we want to go to the bookstore and get a hot chocolate and a novel.

ninety-degree pivot

ShuffleshuffleshuffleshufflepausecheckshuffleSIT

"Would you look at that!"

5:19

"Let's go get breakfast."

GO TO PAGE 212.

He has just fucked me shower-doggy in the SoulCycle stalls. I wanted him and I loved it and the water was warm. How it was supposed to feel the first time. Until I started bawling and slumped to the floor.

He is hunched over me, hands cupping my face, his eyes the color of a glacier as it rolls back into the arctic sea. My breathing catches, then steadies. I have just cried during sex in front of my rapist and I am angry and relieved and humiliated and I cannot face him. I try to look away, but his hands won't let me. I surrender, and smush my cheek into the open space of his palm with a whimper. He holds steady. Worry draws the lines around his eyes, penciled by the kind of attentiveness I was not afforded in our first encounter years before.

I try to speak. I can't. I'm about to lose it all over again when he pulls me into his arms. I sink into him and we fumble, awkwardly, knees knocking against the shower wall, ankles pressed into the thick rubber mat below us. Eventually I am a ball against his chest, and his arms and legs are my protection from the rest of the world. Water, slimed with conditioner, slithers through his leg hair and drains in between us. He is so nice to me and I'm such an embarrassment. The drain gurgles, belches. He rests his head on mine. My heart hurts. I cry.

"I know." He squeezes me, kisses my forehead with the side of his mouth.

"It's ok. I'm here. Shh, shh, I've got you.
I'm sorry.
I'm sorry, baby.
I've got you.
It's ok.
It's ok.
It's ok."

GO TO THE NEXT PAGE.

III.

A Questionable and Poignant Scene Between Our Heroine and an Internationally Controversial Figure

Lights up on JAMES (nonbinary, beautiful, twenty-seven) in a café that overlooks the French Riviera ensconced in light. They fuddle with the teacup in front of them. Enter OSAMA BIN LADEN (six feet four, alive, not what you expect in this moment). JAMES looks up, as if she was expecting company.

*** Note from the playwright: For consistency, JAMES should still be played by Cate Blanchett, Anne Hathaway, or Jessica Chastain. However, if you choose Jessica Chastain, you may want to note in a large gold banner across the stage/screen that reads "THIS IS NOT A SCENE FROM* ZERO DARK THIRTY*" because I can imagine there will be questions. Alternately, if your PR team vetoes this idea, I* *recommend going for a completely different energy in this scene as it exists in liminal space anyhow. Consider season-three-*Gilmore Girls*—era Alexis Bledel, or newcomer and Emmy Award winner Ayo Edebiri. (Despite the fact that she looks nothing like JAMES I am confident she would nail this scene.) Casting OSAMA BIN LADEN is a bit trickier, because you cannot use any of the previous men as they have all been white, and brownface while playing a mass murderer is still brownface. You may want to put out one of those "CASTING" infographics on your Instagram page so you can get submissions from 300+ NYU Tisch hopefuls . . . one of them might be good! You could also contact Ricky Sekhon (who played the role in* Zero Dark Thirty *and famously had no lines in the final edit of the film). Perhaps he would enjoy these lines and be willing to reprise the role. I would recommend conveying our collective recognition that pigeonholing Brown actors into playing antagonists is a racialized trope, and perhaps this could be a two-film contract; one for this role and another for something outside this stereotype that he would be fantastic at and would advance his career. Perhaps we should listen to anti-racism educators and build more opportunities for People of Color to break out of racial stereotypes in our industry if we are also going to cast them within those stereotypes.*

JAMES. Hey, thanks for meeting with me.

OSAMA. Of course, thank you for inviting me.

(They both speak English for some reason, probably because this will premiere in America and whitewashing is what we do best.)

OSAMA. I enjoyed "Love Letter to Osama."

JAMES. What?

OSAMA. Your paper on your professor's theory: "The enemy of my enemy is my friend."

JAMES. You read that?

OSAMA. I did. You had, as the kids say, some points.

JAMES. How did you even get a copy?

OSAMA. Don't worry about that.

(They both stir their tea.)

OSAMA. So, James, why did you invite me here?

JAMES. Well, I thought France would be a good middle ground because obviously you can't get into the U.S. with all the "Top Ten Most Wanted People on Earth" stuff, not to mention the conspiracies you're still alive, and I figured I'd have difficulty getting a visa to Pakistan given the amount of times I searched "how did they do 9/11" in preparation to write this book so—

OSAMA. I don't mean here as in France, I mean here as in meeting with you.

JAMES. Oh. *(Beat.)* I've been thinking about killing my rapist.

OSAMA. Really?

JAMES. Yeah.

OSAMA. That's admirable.

JAMES. You think so?

OSAMA. Yes. I hate rapists. Scum of the earth. Only crime I can think of with no justification.

JAMES. Um, wow? . . . Ok!

OSAMA. *(an inquisitive pause, an eyebrow raised; something to prompt JAMES to continue)*

JAMES. I just wasn't expecting that.

OSAMA. Why not?

JAMES. Oh, I don't know, probably because you're not particularly known for your progressive feminist politics?

OSAMA. I had a lot of wives!

JAMES. That makes you poly, not necessarily progressive. There are a lot of she/theys in Bushwick, for instance, who also think of themselves as progressive feminists when really they're using polyamory unethically as an excuse to avoid accountability in their romantic relationships, which come to think of it doesn't even apply to you because you were polygamous, not polyamorous, a different practice entirely, and the conflation of the two is both anti-feminist and harmful to the radical roots of the latter and—

OSAMA. Fascinating.

JAMES. OK I'M GETTING OFF TRACK, the point is I don't know what to do.

OSAMA. Have you considered flying a plane into the SoulCycle where he works?

JAMES. Actually, yes.

OSAMA. You're having reservations?

JAMES. It would kill so many other people in the process!

OSAMA. I know. That's what I did.

JAMES. Yeah, and I don't necessarily think that was right. Even if your political motivations had, as the kids say, some points.

OSAMA. You're smart.

JAMES. And beautiful, so the boys tell me. ANYWAY, I just don't think mass death will bring me the kind of peace I desire. Did it give you peace?

OSAMA. I had to live in hiding for the next two decades in the mountains of Pakistan, what do you think?

JAMES. That I don't have the same access to wealth, money, or a Pakistani compound so it wouldn't work out as well for me?

OSAMA. I know people—

JAMES. Yeah, I don't—

OSAMA. Some of them are still alive!

JAMES. Which does seem to be a public concern—

OSAMA. Maybe for your rapist.

(Beat. They both laugh.)

JAMES. How did you know my rapist worked at SoulCycle?

OSAMA. Don't worry about it.

JAMES. Did you feel bad? After you did it?

OSAMA. The planes? I didn't do it. I just orchestrated.

JAMES. But didn't you feel guilty about killing all of those people?

OSAMA. I suppose my desire to overthrow American imperialism and do my part to stop the U.S. from annihilating the Middle East was stronger than my compassion for a few people on an aircraft I'd never meet.

JAMES. I mean I also hate American imperialism and how we annihilate the Middle East—

OSAMA. You mean the very imperialism you're complicit in as an American taxpayer?

JAMES. Touché. *(Beat.)* Still, I don't think I could have that kind of tragedy weighing on my conscience. I'm not really going against American imperialism in any meaningful way, just one specific guy.

OSAMA. One specific guy who caused you tragedy and it does not seem to weigh on his conscience.

JAMES. So that means I should just blow up a building?

OSAMA. If you did people might sympathize with your motivations.

JAMES. Who?

OSAMA. Other survivors. Many people who have experienced sexual assault long to see their assailant dead. Arguably, it makes a safer world for them, for other people, and in a world that is built on violence sometimes violence is a natural response.

JAMES. I think that's a quote from one of the Black Panthers . . .

OSAMA. Probably, I didn't come up with it.

JAMES. So the violence is justified?

OSAMA. To some.

JAMES. But to me?

OSAMA. Only you can answer that. It is very possible that if you flew a plane into your rapist's SoulCycle and killed him along with the other thirty to forty people inside you would be jailed, labeled a terrorist—albeit a domestic one—and executed by the state. Years from now, when people will have cooled off enough about the situation, some snappy college twink will write an essay about how the Enemy of Their Enemy Is Their Friend and they will be referring to you.

JAMES. I don't think you can use the word "twink"—

OSAMA. Is it a slur?

JAMES. Are you queer?!

OSAMA. Touché.

JAMES. What's the other possibility?

OSAMA. I hook you up with one of my friends who has a compound in [redacted undisclosed secret location].

JAMES. Yeah . . . that's really nice of you to offer but I don't think that's for me.

OSAMA. Then you have your answer.

JAMES. I'm more confused now than when we sat down. *(Beat.)* Do you think about Christine Hanson?

OSAMA. *(Beat. OSAMA does not move for a moment.)* I think about my own daughters more. *(Another beat.)* Tell me, do you feel the state has protected you as a survivor of sexual assault?

JAMES. No.

OSAMA. In fact, would you agree the state has perpetuated the very rape culture that harmed you?

JAMES. Yes.

OSAMA. So we have something in common: an enemy.

JAMES. Which makes me uncomfortable.

OSAMA. Why?

JAMES: Because you're the villain in so many people's stories?

OSAMA. Yes, but the hero in others'.

JAMES. Just like how my rapist is the villain in mine, but the hero in others'.

OSAMA. Same with Finnegan.

JAMES. How do you know about—?

BOTH. *(in unison)* Don't worry about it.

OSAMA. You've written probably ten thousand words humanizing me, one of the most notorious figures in modern history. There are people reading this book who hate Finnegan and your rapist more than they hate me right now.

JAMES. That's because I'm a good writer.

OSAMA. And because you're stubborn.

JAMES. What the hell?

OSAMA. You are more willing to humanize a man you've never met than a man you once loved and another man who made a mistake because he's human.

JAMES. Oh, so rape is ok because he's human?

OSAMA. No, rape is never justified. I am pointing out that people make grave mistakes, and it sounds like both he and Finnegan made what you would consider grave mistakes. You may not want to hear this, but it does not make them irredeemable people.

JAMES. How the fuck did you become the moral compass of this scene?!

OSAMA. I'm not. I'm saying if you continue down this path your stubbornness may rot into bitterness, and you may be surprised by the outcome.

JAMES. So you do regret it?

OSAMA. I think it is more convenient for you to believe that because if you can see my humanity than you can also see yours.

JAMES. Again, a surprising stroke of wisdom coming from you of all people.

OSAMA. Am I wrong?

JAMES. *(Sighs.)* No, you're not.

OSAMA. I think you have your answer.

JAMES. Or I have fifty more questions.

OSAMA. Sometimes that's the same thing. *(Standing. He is, of course, six feet four.)* Thank you for inviting me to the French Riviera.

JAMES. You're leaving?

OSAMA. I am.

OSAMA heads toward the door, then turns, as if to say one more thing. He doesn't. Perhaps he looks a moment more, then makes his way toward the exit. He vanishes into a projection / special effect that looks like waves on an open ocean.

List of Publicly Available Praise for My Rapist from Assorted Internet Sources:

ClassPass user
4 years After

"[Name] is amazing! I was nervous because I had never taken a class here before but [Name] helped me shake all those first time jitters. Will definitely be back for sure!"

ClassPass user
8 months After

"One of the best instructors at this studio! The beats are always fiyaaaahhhh. I always sweat so much and feel great after. [Name]Nation RISE UP!!!!!!"

Instagram post
3 years After

"50th ride at SOUL!!!! Big shoutout to [Name, Instagram handle] for always pushing me & inspiring me to be my best. Your classes are so hard but you make it fun. So happy to be a part of the SOUL Fam & have found my tribe here. TuesSLAY 4 Lyfe!!"

ClassPass user
2 years After.

"I went to SoulCycle at a time I felt really lost in my life. I won't really go into detail but someone close to me passed away. I was depressed. I had no motivation for anything really. One of my coworkers recommended I try [Name]'s class because they thought he was funny and thought it might lift my spirits. I was resistant because I was like why would this help, you know? It's not gonna bring that person back and I don't really like fitness or exercise or that stuff. Never really been into it. But I went and boy oh boy. It changed me. It really did. My first class I cried and I'm not ashamed to admit that. [Name] is funny like my person was and I didn't think I would laugh like that again. Well, I didn't! At first. But then I did. And it started feeling good again. It took me a long time to go back because it was so emotional for me. But eventually I did and now I'm a regular. It's probably weird to be typing this but maybe someone out there is also depressed and maybe [Name]'s class can help. You don't even have to be a fitness person. I'm not that good at the class but I keep coming because I laugh and feel better. It's my one hour a week where I'm not that sad. His class is great. I'm still not really a fitness person or whatever and I'm not really good, but I come to this class and have been coming for about a year now. I never even miss a week! I didn't believe a place like this could change my life but it did. My life is so much better now. Thanks to [Name]. He really is a great guy."

Reddit user
9 comments down on the responses to "Looking for Good LGBTQ+ Workout Classes in [His City]?" 5 months After

"Honestly I recommend trying [Name]'s class at SOUL on [location]. He is great if you are new and he's super friendly. He also isn't hard to look at! Lol ;)"

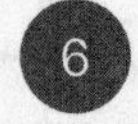

Another Reddit user
10 comments down on the responses to "Looking for Good LGBTQ+ Workout Classes in [His City]?" 9 months After

"your right he rly is sexy!"

His last boyfriend
almost 1 year Before.

"Happy 6 months to my guy. You make me a better person every day. I am so lucky to be loved by you. Can't wait for matching pajamas at Christmas again! :P Love you, [Name]."

Today we have a family meeting about when we are going to kill my grandfather.

Or at least that's what it sounds like, were someone to overhear our conversation.

I am seated at the table as one of his primary caregivers surrounded by the assortment of patriarchs—my father among them—a group I've maintained access to despite being the youngest member and the only one actively growing breasts. I've chosen a baggy sweatshirt today. My nipples hurt. I told my father this, who said, "Well, I think we've got some morphine in the fridge if that'll help?" To which I responded, "Jesus Christ," and we laughed so hard we cried.

Last time we talked about estrogen I cried too. Over breakfast one day he told me that despite everything my face looked different in a good way. I said it could be because I was on estrogen (big reveal!!!) and he asked me how it worked and when I finished Hormones for Trans Femmes 101 he sort of cocked his head to the side and said, "Are you happy?" and I said, "Yes, I am," and he said, "Well then I'm happy too." Later he sent me a picture from my childhood where I had dressed up as Madeline. "This has always been you!" and I knew he was referring to my gender; cue the tears. I seem to always be crying over boys, I admit. I much prefer crying over my father's acceptance of my transness than after bottoming too close to the sun with some guy who makes being uncut his whole personality. When will I learn?

Anywho, apparently the way we're repaying my father for being one of eight trans-affirming dads on the planet is by killing his father because that seems completely fair.

The issue is that he's in pain. We spent the first twenty minutes listening to the patriarchs discuss what a high tolerance my grandfather has. The spine story has been referenced eight times. My grandmother and I look at each other. *WE ARE WOMEN!!!* I send telepathically, which is a stand-in for *WE ALREADY KNOW THIS!!!*

The patriarchs have consulted the folder of documents on the table containing my grandfather's medical papers, insurance plan, power of attorney, doctor's notes, social security card, birth certificates, future funeral arrangements, all of it, soup to nuts. One of them (my uncle) motions to me while another one (my dad) talks.

"Do you want this?" my uncle mouths. I shake my head and lift a palm in protest. I look at my grandmother. *WE ARE WOMEN!!!* Which is a stand-in for *WE KNOW WHAT IT SAYS, WE PUT IT TOGETHER!!!*

The papers from the doctors say what we all know: He won't get better.

The papers from the nurses say what we all know: He is actively getting worse.

The papers from the lawyer say what we all know: He already entrusted money to his family years ago; you have already acquired your inheritances and no one has any incentive to let him die outside of putting him out of his misery.

It's not as cruel as it sounds, letting him die. Which I suppose is different than killing him. Killing is active, whereas letting him die is passive, a sidestep to nature's course. He isn't eating, we have to stroke his throat to coax him to swallow water, he hasn't showered in two days because he doesn't have the energy to sit, he has developed bedsores from sleeping more than the average house cat; this is no way to live. He is essentially nonverbal. His doctors say it's likely the only reason he's alive is because we make it a point to feed him smoothies blended with essential nutrients because he can still manage a straw. If we stop that we will let him die. Kill him, technically, because it's an active choice, but a merciful one. I don't know the ethics, only the outcome.

Some of the patriarchs are hesitant about our plan, probably because they are emotional. (It is their father! They don't want him to suffer! They don't want any of this!) There is arguing, padded with machismo and surprising softness. The arguments are circular. I cleave the cycle:

"One of you once said to me, 'We treat sick dogs better than this,' and from where I sit this is a lot like euthanasia. It's merciful. We don't keep sick dogs around limping about in pain. This man is in so much pain he's being administered morphine, and we can offer him a controlled, dignified, pain-free exit."

They counter that it still sounds like murder, and my grandmother relays the hospice nurse's words: This is an increasingly common practice at the final stage of people's battles with Alzheimer's. The disease is terminal, and force-feeding him to keep him alive carries a cruelty not found in a natural death. We are at an impasse, we have tools in the shape of tiny syringes and electric-blue liquid to make his final days as comfortable as possible. She adds that if we stop feeding him now, under the care of his doctors, we know roughly when he will die. We can prepare, we can be together, we can eliminate the guesswork that has shred our nervous systems and hung them on invisible racks to dry.

The patriarchs are silent, indicating a shift. She has a point, and they know it. *WE ARE WOMEN.*

"Well." My uncle removes his glasses, sharing a look with my dad. "When would we start?"

"Theoretically we could start as soon as today."

The room gradually rebuilds into a smattering of affirmatives but devolves into a clattering of protestations. This week one of them has a big meeting, another one is out of town next week, what if [insert remote relative] wants to be here, one of the wives' schedules needs to be considered. No one has time to kill my grandfather.

I stand. After so long in this house I do have time. "There's never going to be a good time. Death isn't known for being convenient. If we sit here and squabble over schedules we will collectively go as mad as he is and with all due respect, as much as you all come visit and care for him and help us cook when you can, at the end of the day it's the two of us waking him up to suck blended berries from a straw and changing his diapers and washing the sheets at all hours of the night. It isn't fair for everyone to get a vote about this when the outcome of the vote doesn't proportionally affect everyone the same. We're saying we want to do this now. He's ready. He is *trying* to die. We need to let him go."

I have not raised my voice, but they look like scolded children. Perhaps they are. Perhaps it is embarrassing for the one among them growing breasts to be so correct. That is not my issue to sort out. Perhaps I have been a touch harsh. This is their father, after all.

"I get it," I say, returning to my seat and their eye level. "You're losing your dad. I don't want you to have to lose your dad. I don't want to lose my dad some day! But we either stop feeding him this week and we all sit around and celebrate his life and fill his room on his final days with laughter and good food and the knowledge that he was loved, or we relinquish all control and let him pass whenever he will. In the middle of the night or during a nap or by surprise one morning; we won't know. Personally, I'd rather readjust my schedule and be here, and start now."

Silence again. The air crinkles. Someone shifts an elbow. Someone else sips water.

"Alright?" I ask.

"Alright," says my uncle.

"Alright," says my father.

My grandmother nods. Meeting adjourned. Tomorrow, under the care of his hospice nurses we begin starving my grandfather, and in turn, setting him free.

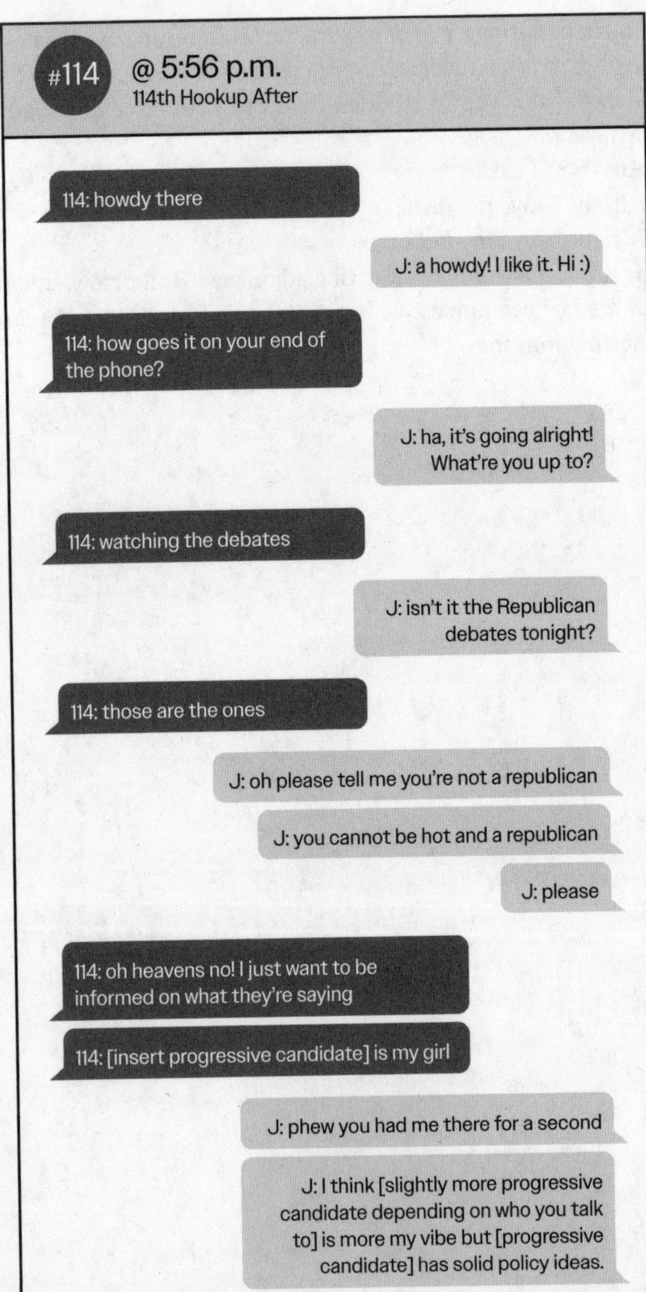
#114
@ 5:56 p.m.
114th Hookup After
114: howdy there
J: a howdy! I like it. Hi :)
114: how goes it on your end of the phone?
J: ha, it's going alright! What're you up to?
114: watching the debates
J: isn't it the Republican debates tonight?
114: those are the ones
J: oh please tell me you're not a republican
J: you cannot be hot and a republican
J: please
114: oh heavens no! I just want to be informed on what they're saying
114: [insert progressive candidate] is my girl
J: phew you had me there for a second
J: I think [slightly more progressive candidate depending on who you talk to] is more my vibe but [progressive candidate] has solid policy ideas.

114: I've had that thought too. I'd absolutely vote for [slightly more progressive candidate] I just think [progressive candidate] has better policy in regards to splitting up these tech companies.

J: yeah I totally agree. I do think [slightly more progressive candidate]'s climate change policies are more thorough and what's the point of splitting up big tech if we're all displaced from natural disasters u feel?

114: I like your brain

J: that compliment just made you ten times hotter

114: I like your smile too

J: well you've got me grinning

114: wanna come over and watch the debates together?

J: do I get to lay on the couch next to you?

114: full transparency I do have a girlfriend, but we are in an open relationship and I would absolutely like to have you on the couch next to me . . . or maybe more? Totally up to you I just wanted you to know everything up front so you could make an informed decision

J: wow, thank you, I really appreciate that! Tbh I wondered if that was your gf in your last post (she's so pretty!) but figured you wouldn't have slid into my DMs if you weren't open lol.

J: are you sure she'd be ok with my coming over?

114: totally! All within the agreements. Just gotta use condoms if it gets there.

J: Great :) because I definitely want to be on the couch with you . . . and you should probably get out the condoms just in case ;)

In our defense we watch thirteen entire minutes of the debates before I kiss him. He looks like Prince Eric if Prince Eric were born in Ohio and had floppy strawberry blond hair and was bisexual. He has this goofy sort of Pixar grin that I make my personal mission to keep constant on his face with my jokes. This means I have to crane my neck from my position as anti-Republican little spoon to measure the effectiveness of my funnies, and eventually I linger looking at said Pixar grin until it is flush against my own, the zipper of my jeans scratching against his.

We make it upstairs to his bedroom, which is surprisingly tidy. "Organization sponsored by Lexapro and insomnia!" He swings his arms wide. Then, questions:

"Can I lay you down on the bed?"

"Can I take your shirt off?"

"Can I touch your dick?"

"Would you like me to get a condom?"

Yes,

Yes,

Yes,

Yes.

Then I am parroting the same inquiries, ogling at his commitment to consent, deciding then and there I'd reward him with doggy. He deserves it.

"Your eyes are rather enchanting." It sounds equal parts marvel and admission coming from him.

"Oh, hush!"

"I'm serious!" He hovers over me, gathering pillows to prop my head. "They're such a deep color. There must be a whole story behind them."

I kiss him. "I like you." I know I can't date him or fall in love with him, neither of which is my intention or desire. Every time I find myself in this position—literally, figuratively—I watch myself fall in what I believe is love, though realistically it is a cocktail of lust, poppers, and grief. Here with #114, I only want to like him. I focus on tying my emotions to reality, engaging with the present. His touch makes me feel fresh, green, revived.

"Good, because I like you too."

The rest of this scene takes place over the course of six hours, oscillating between furious, passionate sex and equally furious, passionate political discussions. At one point we do end up in doggy (success!), my face on its side against the pillow, begging him: harder, deeper, more. As he goes harder, deeper, and more it pushes a sense of pride upstream from belly to heart to mind; I am finally comfortable in this position. Instead of wondering if he, like Finn, no longer wanted to look at me I focus on relaxing my lumbar, and relishing in each stroke. The accompanying ecstasy arches me an inch further and then it happens:

Pain electrocutes my nervous system, then a parade of bullets in my gut. I fall to the sheets with a gasp. By the time I realize what is happening I am shaking and, to my horror, sobbing uncontrollably. My vision is white flashes, my skin sprinkled with sweat. I am midtrigger. #114 must be terrified. I feel him next to me on the bed, but I am facing away, mortified I've burst into full-throated sobs in the heat of intercourse. Snot seeps onto the pillows. I wipe my nose with my finger, wipe my finger on my leg hair, and turn over. I will have to face him eventually.

"I—" I choke. His eyes bleed gray with concern. "I'm so sorry."

His focus darts back and forth between my eyes, searching for the missing pages of the story he saw in them earlier.

"Did I . . ." His voice is tissue soft.

"No, oh god no!" I am regaining my composure. "You didn't do anything wrong. It's just sometimes—" Sometimes I'm like this. Sometimes Finnegan and my rapist win. Sometimes pleasure eclipses me, carved out of reach by the cruel blade of a brain under-resourced. Sometimes the same PTSD that plagues military veterans and sexual assault survivors alike with the same shredded clumps of neural pathways fails me. I cannot contain it. Liquids, shudders, heaves, they burst from me with reckless abandon. I am back to square one, hand over my mouth, wishing I could evaporate.

Gingerly, #114 blankets me with his arms. They feel foreign, delicate, and necessary. His palm flattens between my shoulder blades, and his chest settles next to my ear. The pressure of his body is a cement dam against my ballooning cries, a container to feel pain without the fear I'd disappear altogether. I let myself fill the container. I don't know how long I cry for, I only know his intermittent squeezes, forehead kisses, murmurs of "I'm here, it's ok" are alcohol on my wounds. They sting, they cleanse, they hurt until they don't.

Perhaps it is harder to accept this form of care, gentleness, love when we have been abused, because it puts into perspective the abuse's severity. I am accustomed only to believe I am fuckable, not lovable. I have internalized my brokenness, not my resilience. I am used to Finnegans and rapists and #1s, #2s, #5s, all the way to #113s. #114 is new. #114, whose first instinct is transparency, consent, and to hold me through the discomfort.

I take my first full breath and find a small pool collected in his collarbone, no doubt from my tear ducts. I chuckle. I am humiliated. I am grateful. He strokes my hair, his palm nearly the size of the back of my head.

"James, I am so unbelievably sorry for whatever I—"

"Oh, babe." I touch his cheek. "It wasn't you. Truly, it wasn't you at all." I sigh. I am breathing deeper now. "I guess I owe you a story."

So I tell him. I tell him of Finn and our open relationship and I tell him about my rapist. I tell him of the doctors, the scar tissue, the breakup, my diagnosis. I tell him I had never been triggered like this before, not during sex, not this way, and the way he responded was exactly what I needed and thank you so much, and I'm sorry I became the girl who had a mental breakdown in your bed and I completely understand this was a big story to take in but you seem like such a genuine, caring person and never in a million years would I want you to think you did anything wrong here because actually you did everything right, I am so grateful and whatever version of care or friendship or love this is feels special to me because I don't think I've had this before and I'm sorry I'm crying again?? I promise it won't be as bad this time, I swear.

#114 looks me in the eyes and clears my cheeks with the softest thumb swipes.

"James, I think you're the most beautiful person in the whole world."

I think about the Twin Towers on the way home. #114 showed me an article that my city is considering reverting One World Observatory's name back to Freedom Tower, the very name it replaced in 2009. I think about the presidential debates we barely watched, how many times "freedom" would probably be mentioned, but what an empty word it is. At the same time, I wonder if it's accurate to say this newfound feeling after #114 is freedom.

As a concept, freedom frustrates me, because it has only ever been accessible to those who benefit from the white supremacy that buoys our culture. Even as a beneficiary of many privileges under this system, freedom is still not attainable to me as a survivor of sexual violence. It has been years, and I still cannot find a way to enjoy basic, intimate pleasure with other people. The same culture of white supremacy I benefit from has also harmed me through the perpetuation of a rape culture. The victim-blaming, the legal system, the media, the trivialization and normalization of sexual violence means my story of the back room of the music closet and the midnight in October are more common than not. One of mine just happened to be on 9/11, but it happens to someone, somewhere, every day.

I thumb through the comments on the article, noting how many Arab people consider the renaming an insult, citing the racism and Islamophobia they experienced—and still experience—manufactured by the government in the wake of 9/11. They say the name will never be appropriate until they are free from these oppressions. I "like" each of the comments. As a white person I will never understand their experiences of racism, but the idea of "freedom" coming at the expense of someone else's makes me seethe. The enemy of my enemy is my friend. If freedom has victims it is not true freedom; it is harm in disguise.

I don't think I found freedom with #114. Instead, I think the experience offers me an opportunity to free myself. I ache to be free of Finnegan, my rapist, the flashbacks, the nightmares, the triggers, the suicidal ideation, the black pit in my gut that tells me I am forever broken, forever unlovable. But unlike my rapist, #114 listened to my needs when we hit the crossroads of Rape and Not Rape. Unlike Finnegan, #114 was willing to hold space for my pain instead of discarding me. If my story isn't unique, maybe #114 isn't either.

If it is people who imprison us, it must also be people who set us free. I wonder if freeing myself means finding the #114s instead of dwelling on the Finnegans, the Mr. Andersons, the rapists. I wonder if I'm ready for that.

***

A message:

#114: hi beautiful, text me when you get home?

#114: [redacted phone number].

I save it in my phone. We will become friends. If belonging starts somewhere, I'm starting here this time. In between gentleness and "text me when you get home."

It is Day Three. The front door is now revolving with family members. The patriarchs populate the den most of the time. My cheesecakes have found bellies, the ceiling has found trouble containing the laughter. My grandmother and I dress in what we call "real clothes," which are different than the clothes you wear when you think you may have a direct encounter with the evidence of your loved one's incontinence with regularity.

I have set his midday morphine syringe on the counter as the patriarchs and other assorted family members prattle on about the NCAA—something about Marquette, the Final Four, whatever straight people talk about while their dad dies, I don't know. I crouch to examine the veggie pot pie in the oven when I could swear I hear the sound of wheels rounding the ADA corridor. I wonder if my grandmother is removing the chair from his room for some reason and realize to my horror the reason might be because he's dead. He died, I missed it, and we were all laughing about some stupid game with orange balls and swishy shorts, and he's lying there decomposing and she's taking out the wheelchair because she doesn't know what else to do. Fuck.

"James! Well, hello there, young man!" My former gender has not died, and neither has my grandfather. He is sitting inside the wheelchair, beaming. The room is still with the soundlessness of shock.

"Hello, Grandpa . . ." My oven mitts are frozen midair.

My father claps once and jumps to his feet. "Well, hey there, Pop!"

The rest of the family follows suit with handshakes, back claps, "Wanna watch a little Marquette?" and shuffle the room to accommodate his chair. My grandmother smiles and joins me in the kitchen.

"What happened?" I whisper.

"I don't know!"

He is forming near sentences, pointing to the TV. He looks like he did a year ago. My dad interrupts.

"He said he's hungry?" The words come on a carpet of bewilderment.

"Tell him the veggie pot pie is coming out of the oven, it'll just need to cool . . ."

My dad nods. "I'll keep him occupied."

When my grandfather asks about food for the fifteenth time in as many minutes, I am slicing the pie. I can hear the relief from the men in the room in the form of bright chatter. What a relief to be caught in an Alzheimer's loop instead of the loop around death's door. Death must live on a cul-de-sac.

"I guess we won't need this?" My oven mitt gesticulates to the morphine.

"I guess not." My grandmother surreptitiously empties the liquid into the sink and washes it down the drain with the detachable nozzle.

"And we're going to . . . start feeding him again?"

My grandmother is thinking it, I'm just saying it. "We can't deny him now, can we?"

We can't. This would be killing, not a merciful morphine-sponsored natural ending of life.

She speaks again. "As long as he's awake enough to ask for food I think we should give it to him."

I hand her the plate with warning of its warmth. She thanks me and carefully crosses the room, as if the slightest disruption to its flaky crust would shatter the illusion and my grandfather would disappear back into his comatose slumber.

"Alright!" he exclaims, eyeing the plate. My grandmother looks up at me, and winks. I guess we have more time after all.

I place the oven mitts back in the drawer. Droplets wiggle on the lip of the sink. The athlete on screen shoots a free throw and makes the basket. My grandfather and the rest of the family cheer. I open the fridge, where his daily morphine bundles are banded together like crayons. I want to empty every last one of them, to shock the sink's throat with tubes of medicine rolling through its bowels, so they know he doesn't need them anymore. So they can belch out the pain-free acknowledgment that he's lucid, he's here, he's with us.

I close the refrigerator. He's back, if only for now. We have time.

I take this new time and race up the stairs, to my phone, and rent a car.

No one knows where I'm going, but I've decided to visit my rapist. I have to tell him what he did to me. I need to stop this from happening to anyone else. I am putting my politics into practice. My grandfather is doing well. I have time. This may be the only time I have for a while. My Lyft pulls into the parking lot of the rental car facility.

My grandfather's nurses tell us Alzheimer's is unpredictable, and sometimes this happens. We abandon the plan to let him die peacefully on morphine, and resume feeding him. The patriarchs, each of whom preemptively cleared their schedules this week, remain by his side.

I hand my license to a woman at the counter with perfect plaits and nails as long as her fingers. They click at the keyboard. My heart thunks at my rib cage. I sign paperwork. She hands me the keys.

The patriarchs do not deliberate, they move into a quiet ecosystem of action. My father pulls laundry from one machine and feeds it into the next. My uncle opens a new sponge for my grandfather's bath. My grandmother dries the colander I used for the pasta bake I left cooling on the stovetop.

They all think I am visiting a friend, which isn't a complete lie on the grounds of familiarity. Someone I might still be attracted to. Someone I'm afraid of forgiving. Someone I can't forgive. Someone I'm afraid will remember me. Or won't. The only way to overcome the fear is to go through it. Here I go.

My father assumes cooking duty, taking my place as Commander of the Kitchen, which is really quite fortunate for everyone else as he's an excellent chef. He will use every pot, pan, and skillet in the arsenal and you'll never have the same meal twice, but it will be delicious.

I am in a car. It's a 2022 Kia Soul. It looks like a toaster.

My grandfather eats his son's cooking. He enjoys it.

I plug my destination into my phone and take to the road. I merge onto the interstate.

They sit around the table, plates empty, talking about everything and nothing. They are together.

When night falls, I pull into a rest stop. I don't want to pay for a hotel. I'm not tired, but it's dangerous to drive too long without resting. I don't know why, but I pull up a picture of my rapist on Google Images. Tiny *m*'s. I close the app.

My father wheels my grandfather down the ADA corridor. He lines the wheelchair up with the side of the bed, close enough to where my grandfather can reach the metal handle we attached to the bed years ago.

I stuff T-shirts and flannels into the car windows and spread a sun shield across the dashboard. I pull the hatches on the back seats to flatten them, making a bed through the trunk.

He grabs the silver arc and my father guides him through the reverse pivot before setting him down in bed. He removes my grandfather's house shoes and swings his legs onto the bed so he can lie comfortably.

I ball a hoodie into a makeshift pillow.

He fixes the crowd of comforters around my grandfather.

We sleep.

***

I wake up to windows fogged from my breath. It's early, light is but an idea in the sky's mind, but I know I will not go back to sleep. My foot collides with the trunk door when I stretch my legs. My shoulder is stiff. My bladder is full. I peel open a fresh pair of contact lenses and pop them into their sockets. Cool moisture puckers the car's interior into view. With some difficulty I climb through the space between the front seats, settling behind the wheel, and turn the key in the ignition. I unroll the windows and fold the flannels into a bundle I place in the passenger seat.

My grandmother approaches the bed with my father just steps ahead. My grandfather is awake, but he hasn't said anything yet. My father sits on the edge of the bed, Morning, Pop, how are you feeling, would you like to get up? Eventually there is a nod, an agreement of some sort, and my grandmother goes to fetch the wheelchair.

I reach into the footwell and stuff my feet into my sneakers. I pull the keys out of the ignition and slip them into the pocket of my sweats. They slap with muted metallic thumps against my thigh with each step. I shake my hair from its nighttime bun and jingle toward the bathroom. No one is around. I choose the women's.

Together, my grandmother and my father help my grandfather into his wheelchair. His hair is mussed from a night's sleep, his head droops for a moment, then he lifts it, as if he knows something is supposed to happen next but he can't recall what it is. Do you need to use the bathroom? He responds with something akin to a nod. They wheel him onto the tile where they will transfer him to the toilet.

I fix two sheets of toilet paper atop the seat and sit. The bowl is shallow; I tuck my dick back with my left hand so the tip won't touch the inside. The stream plunks into the water. I exhale. With my right hand I open my phone and check the distance: I am a day's drive away. I thumb over to the SoulCycle website. He is teaching at 8:00 a.m. tomorrow.

My grandfather is working through his second pivot of the day, from wheelchair to toilet. This one is harder, for he must execute it with his pants around his ankles so when he sits he is ready to handle his business. He is holding on to the metal bar we installed in the bathroom years ago, shuffling his feet, not yet positioned to sit, when he grows weary, and with an exhale, begins to urinate.

The only way I will maintain a modicum of control is by visiting him in a public place. Somewhere it would be difficult to rape me. Again. I want our first interaction since the incident to be this one I've prepared for. I don't want to be worried about running into him on the street.

I don't want to keep running into his memory when other men touch me. I want control. I want to get this over with. I want to move on.

Bright yellow liquid hits the tile floor as my grandmother exclaims, Oh, oh! and grabs the handheld plastic urinal in the corner of the bathroom, catching the stream in its opening. He looks at her as if to say he's sorry, then looks away. It's ok, she says. My father, with great effort, holds him upright, forearms hooked under his elbows, eyes looking anywhere, anywhere but down.

I book a bike in the back.

They bleach the floor and wipe.

***

Every so often the road curves before me. The terrain is expansive, boring, flat. It will be like this until I reach his city. Tufts of clouds pass my windshield. The only other car on the road passes me on the right. I toggle the cruise control on. I let my foot relax. I shuffle a playlist.

My grandfather has eaten three orange slices for breakfast, which is not as much as the last day I was there, but still an improvement. It only seems natural his hunger cues would ebb and flow. He laughs at my uncle's joke. Or he laughed because everyone else was laughing. It doesn't matter, he's happy.

"Bloom" by Troye Sivan comes on, and after I roll my eyes I let it play. I wonder where Finn is. Somewhere in a new state with his new husband fucking up a new relationship. Or not fucking it up. Maybe he's very much in love. Maybe that guy was right for him all along and I never was and the fact that they're together now actually has very little to do with me at all. Huh. I ponder.

After the three orange slices my grandfather asks if it's time for bed. My grandmother pretends not to be surprised. He has been awake for forty-five minutes. She says sure, are you tired? Yes, I am! Well then let's get you to bed.

I think about how being raped is the worst thing that has ever happened to me, and how it is the worst thing that has happened to many people. I think about how we, survivors, are hurtling ourselves across highways in small metal contraptions laden with the knowledge someone dehumanized us to the point of indefensible violation. And we just . . . keep going? It baffles me. I think further, and decide being broken up with because I was raped eclipses the rape itself as the worst thing that ever happened to me. If it is unfair to say that I was left because I was raped then I don't know how else to interpret Finn telling me I "just wasn't the confident person he fell in love with anymore."

It doesn't mean anything, my grandmother assures the patriarchs who are hiding their worry under scowls. The doctors said his energy would wane, and that's what's happening right now. Let's give him some rest and see how he feels when he wakes up. They nod in agreement.

I change lanes. I consider the possibility that in order for Finn to knowingly abandon me when I needed him most he must've been relatively broken too. Perhaps he had trauma of his own that was clouding his vision. It is a charitable assumption, but it's possible he did not know how to love me through my own trauma, so he cut himself out of the picture, thinking if he stayed he'd inevitably make it worse. If he told me that at the time I would've never believed him. I would've stuck myself to him like glue out of relentless fear of abandonment or unlovability, which would've only exacerbated the preexisting issues in our relationship. I'm not saying what he did was right, I'm saying it's possible it was kind. The sort of kindness that hurts in the moment. An inconvenient kindness. I flick my blinker and change lanes again.

Lunchtime rolls around. The patriarchs putter about the living room poring over files, fixing sandwiches, stepping onto the back porch for a work call. He hasn't stirred.

I cross into another state, the one that famously birthed my ex-boyfriend. It's appropriately flat and decidedly dismal. It's curious that I've spent considerable time imagining what would happen when

I saw my rapist again, but never imagining my next encounter with Finnegan. I suppose that's because there is a set of expectations for encountering your ex in the wild: an acknowledgment, a hug, a cordial exchange of how are you, you look great, congrats on the wedding, yes, I'm still living in New York, oh that sounds great, I'm happy for you, good to see you, good to see you too, we go on our way. There is no social prescription for encountering an assailant. The unpredictability is the central knot that buoys my anxiety to a constancy, a perpetual gurgle of "what will I do?"

The binary surprises me: I blame Finn and fear my rapist. Probably because one of them professed his love and commitment to me and the other demonstrated considerably more commitment, albeit to his own agenda (much to my detriment). The emotions one might think would be evenly distributed between the two are unilaterally assigned to one or the other: all the anger to Finn, all the excuses for my rapist. All the judgment to Finn, all the curiosity to my rapist. Tears to Finnegan, hyperfixation on my rapist. The assignments are rigid, probably because PTSD is blocking my nervous system from properly filing the memories in my brain.

Intermittently one of them will say something to the tune of "I guess I should go check on him" or "How's Dad doing?" and they meander toward the ADA hallway to investigate, each time to the same finding.

I wonder where Finnegan is. Emotionally, physically, spiritually. I wonder if he regrets how he left things with me. I wonder if he ever thinks of me while he's with his fiancé. I wonder if he ever moved back to New York. A green road sign signaling an exit emerges around the bend. I could stop the car at the next rest stop and unblock him from the internet and find out. I pull the steering wheel to the rhythm of the bend. The exit passes, I keep driving.

He's still breathing. He's fine.

***

I'm driving southwest, half a sandwich in my lap. The Sun burns in the sky.

My grandfather has rolled onto his back. My grandmother says his feet are cold. She pads him with another pair of socks. Outside it is raining.

A plane flies overhead, roaring across the bright swath of blue sky. I must be near an airport.

He's always cold, this is normal, my dad says. Are you sure? He seems colder than usual. My grandmother shakes her head.

My phone dings.

Let him sleep.

It's the app. A man with a rideable mustache, cornrows, and a tattoo ring around his forearm is messaging me about how cute my profile picture is. (I am inclined to agree.) There's no one on the road, so I message him back.

One of the nurses knocks on the door, travel kit in her hand. Her curls are damp.

He's off the next exit, and he's on PrEP. I'm making great time. I need gas anyway.

Routine vitals check, and how are you, Mrs. Rose? Oh, are these your sons!

At the pump I plug in his address. Six minutes. He asks if I want to come be his pillow princess. Yes, I do.

It's so nice to meet you! I see your son—the one with the long hair? I see him—I mean them? Them, yes, I see THEM a lot. Is he here?

Hey, nice to meet you! Thanks for having me over, no I love dogs!! Hellohellohelloohyou'resocute!!! Is she a corgi? Yes, water would be great. This is a cute place, oh, mmmmm, yes of course I want to see the bedroom . . .

No, they're visiting a friend, they'll be back this weekend. Oh that's nice, we all need a vacation! Is your husband sleeping? We'll need to wake him so I can take his vitals. Shall I wake him or would you like to?

His sheets are crisp, like hotel bedding. A Keith Haring copy oversees his bureau. I let him pull my sweats off from where he stands at the foot of the bed. In return he strips, grins, and launches forward.

His blood pressure is down, his heart rate is slower. It is good that he ate! She is encouraged. Have you checked his diaper? No, we have not. Alright, will you help me roll him over? Alright, Mr. Rose, we're going to roll you onto your side.

He flips me belly-down and swallows the top band of the jockstrap in his fist. The other hand rains down on my cheeks with a smack. Good girl. I didn't even have to tell him. I hum with pleasure.

His diaper is full. My grandmother pulls the tabs at his waistline, and together they ball up the soiled bits and remove the diaper. A bedsore blooms on his bottom. The nurse says oh the way one does when they hear someone's pet is missing.

He grabs the lube from his nightstand, dabs some on his finger, and slowly inserts.

She instructs my uncle to grab a tube of cream and a pair of gloves from her kit. He obeys, and she dabs ointment onto the sore.

He spreads my legs from behind with his knees and replaces his finger with the stiffest part of him. He leans forward and saddles his belly in the small of my back. The weight eases any remaining tension in my body. I tell him he can pin my hands down if he wants. Oh yeah, baby girl? Yes, I say, just like tha—oh, YES, just like that.

Fresh diaper in place, the nurse and my grandmother roll him back over. They cover him with a cloud of duvets.
We should tell her about the socks—
What about the socks?
Oh, his feet were rather cold s—
Let me take a look.

We finish, and before I can move he wipes me down with a towel.
Thank you, that's so sweet.
Of course, princess.
He winks, I giggle, he lies back down next to me.

You are certainly right, his feet are extremely cold, she says as she peels off the socks. His skin looks almost gray. Or yellow. Both.

Can I ask you something?
Sure.
Are you a girl? Or are you nonbinary? I don't mean to be rude—
No, it's not rude. I'm nonbinary. But it also feels affirming when I say I'm a trans girl. I like both labels, if that makes sense.
Yeah, it does. He pauses, running the back of his finger across my stubble. I wish I had shaved at the rest stop. I feel self-conscious.
I think you're beautiful, he says. A beautiful nonbinary trans girl. His mustache wings open as he smiles.
His words feel like sunshine, beach waves, chocolate chip cookies straight out of the oven. I am stunned.

Is this normal? My grandmother asks. Instinctively the patriarchs join her. The nurse lifts the hem of his sweatpants to reveal the discoloration has traveled up to his knees. No one says anything for a moment.

If people can be casually cruel that means people can also be casually nice. In an alternate universe I marry this mustache because I am his lovable nonbinary trans girl, but in this universe I feel a calmness that comes from knowing this is where our story begins and ends. This was all I needed. I say thank you, pulling as much warmth as I can muster from his heart as I rise from his chest.

They stand there for a moment, until each of them takes a place on the bed. My grandfather's eyes flit open and closed. It's ok, Pop, my dad says. We're here. Rain pelts the window.

I don't cry, I let the thought beam through me: It can be easy, trans people are beautiful. I didn't need him to tell me that, but I like that he did. I float back to the car, lovability in tow, like gravity on a tool belt, a shield against whatever will happen at SoulCycle tomorrow morning.

When my father calls me, I answer on speaker.

"Hey, Dad!"

"Hey, James." He sounds quiet.

"Are you ok?"

"Yeah." Then a pause. My face drains. I know what he's about to say. "Will you pull over for a second?"

They told stories while he died. Stories about his childhood and their childhood and the houses they grew up in. They talked about the sports they played and how he met my grandmother and showed him pictures of Appalachia when he was awake and once he even smiled at them. Like a Funeral Pregame, but with less planning.

Every now and again he would seem to come to and ask where he was and they would explain he was at home, who they were, that they loved him, that he was safe, that everyone would be ok. And he would nod off on a ribbon of "oh, oh, oh yes, that's right." At one point in some strange bolt of lucidity he said, "Where the hell is James?" and everyone laughed because it was the one time I wasn't there and I was the one person he remembered and when my dad told me he was afraid I'd be upset but I laughed and laughed because it was ridiculous and ironic and perfect. Where the hell is James. James was being fucked inside a condo somewhere in a flyover state by a man whose name she doesn't even know. No, scratch that. James was experiencing pleasure. James was experiencing gender euphoria. Where the hell was James? Patching up her heart, fixing their brain, being lovable, not crying. James was doing well.

My dad said they were doing ok. They had cried, for a little bit, and then they stopped. I told him I was sorry he was gone. My dad said he wasn't sorry because he's been gone a long time. He said it felt like a weight had been lifted. He said he felt peace. I said I almost felt guilty for feeling the same. We decided death isn't always sad. Sometimes it's just a release. Or a relief. Both.

He told me that as my grandfather was dying it was raining, and they all huddled around him and held his hands. He told me they heard a sound, and they all looked toward the window. There on the sill, all wet and scraggly, were six red birds. They stayed and watched until the comforter no longer moved up and down with his breath, and then, just like that, they flew away.

***

I don't know how long I've sat on the shoulder of the interstate, two hands on the wheel, seatbelt on, not moving. I've deflated over missing my grandfather's death because I was getting fucked by a man whose name I don't know, tempering this regret with a slew of reminders:

It wasn't my fault, blame was useless, we thought we had time, and I was trying to prioritize myself—myself? Or my rapist? I'm not sure. It's hard to say. It unspools every time I run it through. I think about the last time I talked to my grandfather, how I told him I loved him, how he held my hand and didn't let go. I think about how the rest of my family watched him turn cold and pale and heard him death rattle, and I decide I'm grateful that was not my final memory.

Eventually I unbuckle and crawl out the passenger door. I stumble into a field of yellow grasses and instinctively lift my hands toward the sky and bellow. It feels fantastic. I bellow again. I don't know if I'm saying words or if I'm reduced to sounds, I only know whooping and screaming and shaking my body and jumping up and down and pumping my arms wildly gets it out. Whatever it is I am discharging it, I am freeing myself, I am loosening, lightening, releasing. When I tire, I sit in the grass. The sky promises darkness, and soon.

From the open door I hear my email ding. I crawl back to the driver's seat and pick up my phone.

YOU'RE CONFIRMED: SOULCYCLE TOMORROW AT 8:00 A.M.

I check the drive time.

Where the hell is James?

I put my hands on the steering wheel and look to my left. A cleft in the median is feet ahead of me, guarded by a white rectangle that reads "AUTHORIZED VEHICLES ONLY." On this side of the median: the road to the neon signs, latticework, ponytails, black shorts, headsets, SoulCycle, the same cycle, the same loop. On the other side: the road to my city, my estrogen pills, a notebook, a therapist, EMDR, my family, survival, control, trusting my body, home.

I put the key in the ignition. It snags on the windshield-wiper control. The windshield wipers begin frantically squeaking across the dash. It startles me. I laugh, I turn them off. I turn the key and begin driving. The Sun looms in a sky she painted pink, sinking into her artwork, looking over her shoulder at me. At the last second, I yank the steering wheel to the left and shoot through the unauthorized-vehicle opening.

I point the car home, and I floor it.

Notes

9 *You know exactly which Joanne . . . :* bell hooks, *The Will to Change* (Washington Square Press, 2004), 52–53. hooks critiques Harry Potter and by extension its author for "reinscribing patriarchal masculinity . . . racism, imperialism, and sexism."

42 *The three stages as outlined . . . :* Johns Hopkins University, "Stages of Alzheimer's Disease," https://www.hopkinsmedicine.org/health/conditions-and-diseases/alzheimers-disease/stages-of-alzheimer-disease.

42 *The seven stages as outlined . . . :* Alzheimer's Caregivers Network, "Understanding the 7 Stages of Alzheimer's Disease," https://alzheimerscaregivers.org/the-7-stages-of-alzheimers/.

50 *shot him in front of his kids:* John Friedman, "Navy SEAL Rob O'Neill Recounts bin Laden's Death," National September 11 Memorial & Museum, https://www.911memorial.org/connect/blog/navy-seal-rob-oneill-recounts-bin-ladens-death.

50 *"Like, his daughter was there . . .":* Nicholas Schmidle, "Getting Bin Laden," *The New Yorker*, August 1, 2011, https://www.newyorker.com/magazine/2011/08/08/getting-bin-laden.

50 *Sixty million dollars' worth . . . :* While the exact price is unknown to the public at the time of this book's publication, a general cost can be inferred looking at the unit costs listed here: https://odin.tradoc.army.mil/WEG/Asset/UH-60L_Black_Hawk_American_Utility_Helicopter/1000.

50 *Average salaries of $54,000 . . . :* "A SEAL's Salary: Typical Navy SEAL Makes About $54,000," ABC News, May 4, 2011, https://abcnews.go.com/Business/osama-bin-laden-navy-seal-team-raided-obamas/story?id=13517776#:~:text=Some%20up%20to%20six%20figures%20depending%20on%20skill%20set.&text=May%204%2C%202011%20%E2%80%94,off%20such%20a%20risky%20mission%3F.

51 *Four-Tube night vision goggles . . . :* Amanda Macias, "The Secret Night Vision Goggles SEAL Team Six Wore on the Bin Laden Raid," *Business Insider*, June 2015, https://www.businessinsider.com/the-secret-night-vision-goggles-seal-team-six-wore-on-the-bin-laden-raid-2015-6.

51 *An entire life-size model . . . :* Barack Obama, *A Promised Land* (Crown Publishing Group, 2020), 680.

51 *Penicillin shots . . . :* Drugs.com, "Penicillin g Potassium Prices, Coupons, Copay Cards & Patient Assistance," https://www.drugs.com/price-guide/penicillin-g-potassium.

51 *There was also a dog . . . :* Schmidle, "Getting Bin Laden."

51 *crashed one of their little planes . . . :* Schmidle, "Getting Bin Laden."

52 *Another fun fact is . . . :* Schmidle, "Getting Bin Laden."

52 *They also shot Osama . . . :* Ryan Pickrell, "Obama Thanked Navy SEAL McRaven for Overseeing the bin Laden Raid by Gifting Him a Tape Measure," *Business Insider*, May 2, 2021, https://www.businessinsider.com/obama-gifted-bin-laden-raid-navy-seal-a-tape-measure-2020-11.

52 *And then the Navy SEAL . . . :* Obama, *A Promised Land*, 682.

53 *When they all got home . . . :* Walter Napier III, "Operation Neptune Spear: 10 Year Anniversary," Nellis Air Force Base, April 30, 2021, https://www.nellis.af.mil/News/Article/2591901/operation-neptune-spear-10-year-anniversary/.

54 *Last fun fact I swear:* "Bin Laden's Not-So-Customary Burial," PBS News, May 3, 2011, https://www.pbs.org/newshour/world/bin-ladens-not-so-customary-burial

77 *"weapons of mass destruction":* Dick Cheney interview, *60 Minutes*, November 14, 2001, https://georgewbush-whitehouse.archives.gov/vicepresident/news-speeches/speeches/vp20011114.html.

80 *he circumvented the small bathroom:* "California Man Sentenced to Federal Prison for Assaulting Child on Aircraft," press release, U.S. Attorney's Office, Middle District of Florida, September 27, 2023, https://www.justice.gov/usao-mdfl/pr/california-man-sentenced-federal-prison-assaulting-child-aircraft.

118 *"I think they've taken over the cockpit":* "Extract: 'We Have Some Planes,'" BBC News, July 23, 2004, http://news.bbc.co.uk/2/hi/americas/3919613.stm.

119 *donated it to the 9/11 museum:* Jan Seidler Ramirez, "New on View: Youngest 9/11 Victim's Stuffed Peter Rabbit," National September 11 Memorial & Museum, https://www.911memorial.org/connect/blog/new-view-youngest-911-victims-stuffed-peter-rabbit.

120 *"She put stickers on everything . . . that did this awful murder":* Elizabeth Chuck, "Christine Lee Hanson, Youngest 9/11 Victim, Remembered as a 'Really Special Little Girl,'" NBC News, September 8, 2021, https://www.nbcnews.com/news/us-news/christine-lee-hanson-youngest-9-11-victim-remembered-really-special-n1278730.

120 *I am angry that 81 percent . . . :* National Sexual Violence Resource Center, 2018, https://www.nsvrc.org/statistics.

121 *"It's getting bad, Dad":* "Extract: 'We Have Some Planes.'"

Acknowledgments

I fucking LOVE acknowledgments and I am not going to be brief about mine! I am eternally grateful to have a massive village of people who knew just how insane I am / this book would be and said yes, let's make this happen. Experimental writing is a difficult sell these days—especially as a debut—and it is not lost on me what a privilege it is to be published. If you are reading this, you are a part of making this dream of mine come true, and I wish I could buy you all the ethically sourced deluxe electric vehicle of your dreams.

In between performances of *Cabaret* I cold emailed Mollie Glick and said, "I think you're the only person in the industry cool enough to represent this book." Thank you to Via Romano for forwarding her that email while she was on vacation and saying something to the tune of "This girl is nuts but I think she can write." (I'm paraphrasing, but you get the gist.) Via, thank you for believing in me. Mollie, thank you for pointing to your bookshelf and saying, "You belong here." I cried in the elevator; it is the moment every author dreams of. Thank you for championing me, mentoring me, welcoming me into this world. You are simply the best.

Thank you to the rest of my fabulous CAA team: Jamie Stockton, Kathryn Driscoll, Jennifer Simpson, Ali Ehrlich, and Kate Childs.

Thank you to my tremendous team at Avalon Artists: Craig, Ashley, and Jack, who kept my theater career running while I was typing away.

At an afterparty I looked to my left and saw someone with pink hair and complimented their outfit. That turned out to be Sarah Robbins, my fabulous editor. Thank you for reading Section II on a laptop at 7:00 p.m. in the office with the lights out. Thank you for calling me from another state to say, "Actually the book is good, just fix these fifty-six things." Thank you for answering my unprompted FaceTimes. Thank you for solving all the problems I couldn't.

To the rest of my exceptional team at Abrams: Lisa Silverman, Sarah Masterson Hally, Eli Mock, Ruby Rosenfeld, Logan Hill, Carolyn Levin, Taryn Roeder, Stephanie Keane, Melanie Chang, and everyone else who worked on this book after we had to send this page to print.

Thank you, Haley Jakobson, who said, "You're next." Thank you, Distinctly Sapphic, who held it first. Thank you, Nic Marna, who heard most of this out loud on FaceTime, and the Not OK Girls: Allison Billmeyer, Calista Ginn, Callan O'Neill, Carly Croman, Catherine Merritt, Catie Davis, Gillian Halper, Gracie Jenkins, Jeanne Cassiers, Kelly Cutchin, Liv Sherman, and Vanessa Bride. Your comments, your care, and your criticism made me a better writer. Your friendship makes me a better person.

Thank you: Marian Schembari, for the advice. Charlotte Shane, whose Bad Advice from Bad Women made me want to write again. Zachary Zane and Eli Rallo, for your help early on. Jacob Tobia, for the late-night laughs across the country. Randi and Gaël, who helped me out of the darkest moments.

Thank you: Victoria Beaudoin, for knowing me before and through it all. Ali Funkhouser, for the undying support. Katie Spelman, for the memes. Eva Reign, for reminding me joy is resistance. Becky Whitcomb, for the PowerPoints. Shohreh Davoodi, for Detroit-style pizza adventures. Michael Glavan, for your gentleness. Cecilia Gentili, for your guidance.

Thank you, Zach Burmeister, for letting me read my sex life to you all too many times, for the engraved editing pen, and the giant table in your kitchen where I finally figured out Section II. As I write these acknowledgments we are sitting on your roof and you are reading a self-help book (good, keep reading). Our friendship means the world to me. I will know I've made it as an author when one of your twinks looks at your bookshelf and says, "Omg I love that one!" and it's mine :)

Thank you, Jordan Underwood, for the best T4T friendship I'll ever know. You FaceTimed me in the middle of writing this sentence and I lost my train of thought because we talked for hours, as we always do. Every moment we spend together makes me whole. Thank you for yelling at me, crying with me, pushing me, believing in me, driving me home. Thank you for loving me, even when I didn't deserve it. I love you. And thank you, Jess Lopez, for telling me I have amazing tits. They're almost as good as yours.

Thank you to my mom, who put me in the library before school because she knew I loved to read, who always said, "You're going to write a book one day," for keeping the first one I ever wrote. Thank you to my dad, for reading to me my entire life, for printing out my first online book review when I was fourteen, for fielding the hardest phone call after that midnight in October. Thank you to D, the most creative wordsmith in the family, who taught me how to create art. To my sister, for AP Christmas. To my favorite brother in the whole world, who somehow managed to put up with all this. I am so proud of who we've become as a family. Thank you for showing me love is easy, and being the first place I came to heal. Love you to the moon and back.

Thank you to my uncle, for his service, and to my aunt, for taking me to the city first.

Thank you to my grandmother, the true writer of the family, who made me a feminist and a thinker. Your story inspires me every day. I love you, air buckets.

Thank you to my grandfather, for taking me to the bookstore every visit. I brought your book with me every day to write this so you could be with me. I love you. Rest easy.

Thank you to everyone on my corner of the internet. Some of you have been there since that night in October, holding my hand through this. It is your stories that kept me going. It is your DMs I carry with me—many of which I etched into the border of the proposal to publish this book. You have truly been with me every step of the way. I firmly believe we heal in community, and I feel incredibly lucky that you are part of mine. Thank you for showing me the internet can be a place to connect, to seek comfort, to grow together. Thank you for reminding me that when given the choice, people want to help, to be good to each other, to heal. If I could stand on a street corner and give each of you the warmest, consensual hug of your life I would do it.

To every survivor, I love you. I hope one day we live in a world where a book like this is unfathomable, for we are free.